Club Game

Books by Aaron Sleazy

Sleazy Stories: Confessions of an Infamous Modern Seducer of Women

Debunking the Seduction Community: The Exposition of a Sham Industry and a Primer on Seducing Women

Minimal Game: The No-Nonsense Guide to Getting Girls

Johnny's Journey: Critical Lessons from my Involvement with the Seduction Community (ed.)

Club Game: The No-Nonsense Guide to Getting Girls in Clubs and Bars

In German:
Schmierige Geschichten: Bekennntnisse eines modernen Verführers

Club Game

The No-Nonsense Guide to Meeting Women in Clubs and Bars

Aaron Sleazy

To Hank

Contents

Preface

Clubs and bars are a source of never-ending frustration for many men. Weekend after weekend they go out, spending many hours and plenty of money, only to get virtually nothing in return. The image of clubs in advertising, music videos, or on the Internet home pages of clubs themselves has little to do with reality. On pictures it's all about beautiful people, and the promise of easy sex. Few men, and even fewer women, would openly say that they primarily go out because they hope to get laid. Yet, this particular goal is nonetheless high on their list. Most men don't really know how to reach it, though, which is reflected in phrases like "getting lucky". Luck does play a role, but you can increase your odds significantly. In this book I will show you how.

In fact, the odds are pathetically low for most guys. One might legitimately ask what the issue is, given that there are so many seemingly willing women around. A main cause of this problem is that people who don't go out regularly, and even many who do, don't quite understand how clubs work, on both a sociological and psychological level. I will cover those areas in great detail, but don't worry, *Club Game* is far from being a dry academic exercise. Quite the contrary, it draws from my extensive experience.

I may have been a statistical outlier, considering that most people don't seem to get laid an awful lot from going to clubs and bars. Yet, all the possibilities are there. Girls certainly wouldn't doll themselves up if they only wanted to hang out with all their girlfriends. Night clubs make for a poor socializing environment due to noise and, normally, an excess of visual stimulation. If girls didn't want to get laid, they would stay at home and play board games with their friends.

Club Game is intended to bridge the gap between your expectations and reality. If you are at a complete loss and every time you hooked up with a girl it just happened and you didn't know how you did it, or because you were simply drunk, then you will learn a few things from this book. I won't promise that you'll get laid every night if you follow my advice. However, I would be very surprised if you didn't end up having more success with women as a consequence. Girls really are going out to meet guys — guys like you.

Aaron Sleazy

Acknowledgements

This book had a long gestation period. It all began with an invitation to give a seminar on club game in Oslo in 2008. This led to more seminars in Europe and the United States, but eventually life caught up with me, which meant that I had to put *Club Game* indefinitely on hold a total of three times. This book has existed as a draft for over half a decade, since it essentially was a byproduct of the preparation of my first seminar.

Without the help of some people *Club Game* certainly would never have happened. Arguably the most important role was played by Terry who introduced me to the alternative nightlife scene in London. I wasn't overly fond of mainstream clubs, but he showed me that night clubs can actually be a source of great fun, and not just because of the women. He also taught me how dress to get laid more easily. It was the starting point of something great.

Soon afterwards, I began posting stories of my adventures online, and the responses I received were motivation enough for me to keep writing. People felt that my insights were quite unusual and helped them to solve some of their problems with women. Some of those guys kept emailing me in irregular intervals ever since I hinted that I was working on a book on club game. Those reminders were much appreciated as well.

The few seminars I've given on club game also shaped the content of the book. I'd like to thank the organizers and attendees for making them possible. I furthermore would like to thank the attendees for their questions and feedback, which is directly reflected in this book. I also would like to thank the regulars on both my forum and blog for the fruitful exchanges I've had with them.

As *Club Game* was nearing completion, I received constructive feedback from a number of friends and followers. I would like to warmly thank, in alphabetical order, Assanova, Illuminatus, Isidia, Kriminal, and TheLetter for the time they've taken to read drafts, and send me their extensive notes. Furthermore, I would like to thank Corley Atherton for doing a great job at editing this book. He has been actively involved for the last two years.

Preparation

Preliminaries

Overview

Club Game is divided into two parts. The first part, Preparation, gives an outline of seduction, and highlights a number of important foundational steps. It is intended for guys who need a bit more help to get started. I mainly focus on how you can set yourself apart from your competition and maximize your chances of success. Don't worry, I won't make you wear feather boas, plateau boots, and night-vision goggles. The three chapters Preliminaries, Foundations of Success, and Getting the Edge should be viewed as one unit, and read from beginning to end.

Those of you who consider themselves to be doing pretty okay with women may want to either skim those three chapters, or skip ahead to the second part of this book, Party. In that part I focus on the finer details of club game. Note that I often mention clubs when I mean clubs and bars. The distinction is often arbitrary anyway, since many bars have small dance floors, or charge for cover. Some are small clubs that only call themselves bars for marketing purposes, it seems.

In the chapter Club Sociology I present a high-level description of the dynamics in clubs. Many guys are oblivious to those. In short, I want you to learn how to discover clubs in your city that will make it easier for you to meet girls. This segues into the chapter High-Level Strategies, where I reveal effective methods for planning your night. Good preparation on that front will pay off handsomely.

The chapter Meeting Women is about the mindset and behavior of women you meet on your nights out. As you may know, they act quite a bit differently than during the day. A particular focus is on how to chose a woman to approach. An experienced guy will approach only a small handful of women, if at all, and have a very good chance of getting laid. Once you've decided which woman to approach, you may want to know how to approach effectively, which I discuss in the chapter Successful Approaches. This has very little to do with what proponents of the mainstream seduction community, so-called pick-up artists (PUAs) teach.

Once you've successfully approached a girl, you should focus on getting laid with her. The chapter Taking Action is about that. You will learn effective strategies that will dramatically cut down the time you need to get your dick wet.

I'm making the assumption that you, dear reader, are

male and interested in women. I also assume that you have some experience with women. There is no point in me telling you how great clubs are, and how easy it is to meet girls there if you hardly know what it's like to kiss a girl, or if you get nervous when a girl looks at you, let alone attempts to flirt with you.

In short, you should feel reasonably comfortable around members of the opposite sex. You should also be somewhat comfortable meeting girls, and know how to lead an interaction all the way to the bedroom. If you need two or three dates for that, that's fine. I'll then teach you how you'll get there much faster. On the other hand, if you have hardly any experience with women, then this book is probably not yet suitable for you. In that case I recommend you have a look at my book *Minimal Game* first, which is a basic guide to meeting girls.

You will get more out of *Club Game* if you happen to live in a big city. The downside, though, is that you will have to make a bigger effort to set yourself apart from the crowd. In smaller cities the nightlife is often less exciting, but there is also much less competition. Take your situation into account as you go through this book. This doesn't mean that the advice in this book doesn't apply to smaller cities. People may be a bit more uptight, but girls are girls regardless.

Big city life

I spent a good two years living in central London, so I
can't help but wax lyrical about how great night clubs in
great cities can be. London has an amazing night life,
unmatched by any other city I've ever been to. In most
cities you are either a so-called hipster or mainstream,
but in London people can play much more diverse roles.
This is also reflected in the crowds some venues attract.
It's part of a chicken-or-egg problem. Probably you first
have someone putting on a club night, which they subse-
quently refine to meet the taste of the crowd they want to
attract. If you go out in London you will quickly notice
that there are not only different kinds of women in different venues, but also that some districts have a quite
distinct feel to them. Let me therefore take you on an
imaginary ride through the city.

You start out in the West End and you bump into people
in preppy clothes. Choosing a more upscale venue, you
notice men with too much spare change who are eager
to blow it on bottle service. Looking around, it's obvious
that the women in those places dress in a similar style.
You've got the banksters in their Savile Row suit, and
young women who have maxed out their overdraft for a
Chanel dress and Christian Louboutin shoes. Of course
they now need a guy to rebalance their bank account.

Because this almost institutionalized form of prostitution
irks you, you then head north to Camden, where you are
surrounded by Pete Doherty and Russell Brand looka-

likes, while the women celebrate heroin chic, but it's not clear how much of it is an act. It's all about rock music and getting wasted. You unsuccessfully try to get into Koko, an enormous club catering to that crowd. Sadly, you look as if you've got a day job, so they tell you to get lost.

Disillusioned, you catch the next cab and tell the driver to drop you off somewhere where you can have a drink in a civilized manner. Because you don't look like the kind of guy who feels comfortable in a hard rock bar, and he lacks creativity, he drops you off in front of a Walkabout pub. You swing open the front door, and what do you see? A loud mob of rugged guys. You plunk down at the bar and have a lager. As you look around, you can't fail to notice the many rather athletic and seemingly unintellectual girls in the crowd who fawn over the guys with the biggest pectorals.

Suddenly two young things bump into you, ending up hanging on your neck, and slur that you look cute. The next thing they say is that they accidentally ended up in the wrong place, and ask whether you'd like to share a cab with them to go somewhere nicer. As the three of you hop into the cab, it slowly dawns on you that in their drunken state they have mistaken you not for the blowhard you are, but somehow believe you tried to pull off an ironic hipster style by wearing a tight suit. Your lack of irony is completely lost on them. They consequently help you to further improve your outfit by putting fake flowers in your hair. Then the other girl straddles you as she applies eye-liner on you. Now you fit into the hipster crowd in Shoreditch, where they celebrate carnival every weekend and seemingly everything goes.

This description is not as much of a caricature as you may think. While I haven't had a night exactly like that, I've experienced all these things, and many more. The point of this collection of recollections is not to brag how awesome my life in London was. Sure, the partying was great, fantastic even, but the point I'm trying to make is that if you haven't spent much time going out, or just go to the same places over and over, then you don't know how incredibly varied the nightlife can be. You may not even be aware of the fact that it's usually particular groups who chose to hang out in particular venues.

Benefits of clubs

There are many ways to meet women. You could try your extended social circle, hit on co-workers, go to public events, or check out the girls you meet through your hobbies. Online dating is also very common. However, for a young man living in a reasonably large city, bars and night clubs offer the by far most efficient way to meet women. The main reason is that those venues allow you to potentially meet a large number of mostly young women, and therefore sexually more desirable ones, within a very short amount of time. Further, the women are preselected, because those who think they have a hard time competing for men won't even bother going to clubs. The result is that in one night in a busy club you are exposed to more attractive women than you meet at work or through your friends during an entire year.

Clubs are designed to facilitate sexual encounters. One night stands are common, and what initially started out as a mere one-night stand can easily evolve into a fling or a long-term relationship, if this is what you are interested in. In my opinion, sexual attraction plays a very important role in a relationship, which is why I recommend having sex with a woman as quickly as possible, and afterwards decide how much you like her. Otherwise you may find that the woman you thought you would be oh-so compatible with is a world-class expert in making you lose your erection due to her utter lack of passion or sub-par technical ability in the bedroom. If you haven't had sex with a woman, you don't know her. Only afterwards will she start to reveal her true self.

It seems that it's a lot easier to have a one-night stand than to get a date. Especially for the post-college and professional crowd in big cities, going on a date is a significant time commitment, which women don't take lightly. Getting ready and meeting up for a date amounts to at least two hours. This implies that if you do go on a date, you've got a very good chance to get laid if you don't do anything stupid. On the other hand, if you meet a woman in a nightclub, then she's dolled up and, well, in the club already. Going home with someone she

met in the club doesn't require any further time investment. Whether she goes home alone or takes you with
her won't make much of a difference to her schedule.
But compare this to meeting her during the week, when
a date fills out an entire evening, with or without sex! In
the worst case she may not even have time to have sex
with you because she has to get up early the next day for
work.

Online dating is also popular. Better-looking men and
those who enjoy high monetary status may find it com-
parably easy to meet women through dating sites. Yet,
from what I hear from people who pursue online dating
systematically and successfully, you can also waste a lot
of time. It's not uncommon that you email women, send
text messages, talk on the phone, or exchange pictures.
But then you meet her, and quickly realize that her pictures were five years old or digitally manipulated. Even
worse, sometimes you may get along great on the phone
or in email conversations, only to find out that there is
absolutely no spark between the two of you.

Now compare this with the option of going to a night
club you enjoy, listening to great music, maybe meeting
up with some of your friends, *and* getting laid on top
of that! In clubs women are all around you, and you
can decide for yourself whether you like them or not.
There is no need to ask yourself whether she might look
as good in real life as on her pictures, because real life is
happening right in front of you.

Let me discuss one important point people occasionally

bring up. There is the belief that you can't meet a suitable partner for a long-term relationship in a nightclub, or that night clubs are shady if not downright sleazy places. They also fantasize that all women are sluts and host to countless STDs. In conservative environments such resentments may be common, but I would view it as questionable if a single woman said she never goes out. She's either lying, or maladjusted.

Clubs and bars are sociable places. Even though they facilitate quick sexual encounters, they are also places where people hang out. Of course, people hang out in clubs and bars instead of sitting around someone's kitchen table to some degree because they hope to meet someone to have sex with. I'd like you to keep this in mind because it implies that if you *only* go to clubs to get laid you miss the point. I also doubt that you'll be successful in a place you don't enjoy, since it is obvious to others if you're only there for the women.

Realistic expectations

Before we dive in, I would like to give you a brief overview of my view on seduction, which you may be familiar with from my book *Minimal Game*. You will find that it is rooted in reality instead of fantasy. I tend to be blunt, and if you are the kind of person who is quick to interpret statements that are true but not politically correct as a threat to your self-image, then you are likely to get upset a few times. In this case please calm down, take a deep breath, and re-read the offending passage the day after.

The main idea behind the method of seduction I advocate is that picking up women and seducing them is neither about manipulation nor deception. You cannot make a woman interested in you by using fancy pickup lines or pretending to be someone you are not. The word *seduction* itself is quite a misnomer since it's not so much the case that the man seduces the woman. Both have to work together to make it happen, even though it's normally the man's job to move the interaction forward all the way to sex. As you will learn through experience, you can get sexual with women within a relatively short amount of time, and this is only possible when there is mutual sexual attraction.

Romance, especially the kind of romance that is promoted in mainstream media, is reserved for losers. You may think that you have to take her out to a fancy restaurant, theater, or movie, and that the earliest time to attempt to kiss her is at the end of the first date. In reality, though, she will act on her impulses if she meets a man she finds attractive. She can of course be attracted to the guy who follows the traditional dating routine, but in this case the fancy dinners were optional and she would have been happy to have sex with him right away.

Financial and social status do tip the scales. If you are pursuing one-night stands in clubs, this is less of an issue. Women focus on signals that can't easily be faked when assessing prospective sexual partners. This means that if she thinks you are hot, you are in a better position to get her than some other guy who may only pretend to have money but isn't quite so good-looking.

Most people who are gainfully employed can fake to have more money than they really do. You might have guessed that this is the reason why some women stick to a protocol that prescribes three mandatory dates and minimal sexual contact, because in order to assess whether you are a proper walking wallet, she has to make you spend money on her. But don't get too hung up on those realities of life. If she's into guys because of their money, she isn't necessarily sexually attracted to them. You can meet quite a few bored wives of successful professionals in clubs who are craving for some excitement and stimulation while hubby is on yet another business trip.

But how do you get laid then if you don't want to spend money and risk being taken for a ride? The surprisingly simple answer is that cool guys get laid, and always got laid. Therefore you just have to become a cool guy. Don't laugh! There is an undeniable kernel of truth in this flippant statement. It's not so difficult to become a cool guy. My total investment in London amounted to £200 for a new wardrobe and spare change for cover charge. Money can make it easier, but spare time is a much bigger factor. Spare time is even important if you normally get girls due to status and money. If you spend more time on meeting girls, you should notice that your sex life improves considerably.

Rapid improvement

I believe, based on my experience, that going out on your own is the fastest way to improve, and I suggest you try it yourself. This doesn't mean that you can't talk to anybody, or that you can't bump into friends and acquaintances in the venue. Further, you certainly don't have to go out on your own all the time. Instead, make it a habit to go out on your own at least every once in a while, so that you put yourself outside your comfort zone. By doing so you actively decide how your night out will develop, with the first step being that you decide where you want to go. It is all too easy to fall into a passive role when going out with friends. In the following, I'm addressing a reader who is not yet comfortable going out on his own. However, if you are, then please skip ahead to the next chapter, Foundations of Success.

Going out on your own and hitting on girls isn't a big deal — until you try doing it and freeze up. A timid character might find this initial step in the interaction daunting. Should this apply to you, then you probably have to work on some aspects of your personality. There is no way you will quickly turn from being a complete pushover most of your waking life into someone who effortlessly pulls girls home from the club. At the very least, you will have to learn how to take the initiative, but you also have to stop thinking about what all the other people who don't know you and don't care about you might think about you. They really don't care about you.

Repeated exposure works very well. As so often in life, there is no gradual introduction. It's not as if you can go out a little bit on your own, or kind of hit on a girl. Don't kid yourself! She knows that you're expressing sexual interest when you ask her how she's doing, in some seedy night club at 2 a.m. You are either out on your own, or with friends, or not at all. Likewise, you either hit on a girl, or not. Also, please stop lying to yourself and pretend that you weren't really interested in her if she shot you down. If you weren't interested in her, then why did you bother talking to her in the first place?

You will have to push yourself. Do your homework and make sure you look the part — more details are to be found in subsequent chapters of this book. Then, pick a club for next Friday or Saturday, and decide to go there. From there on it's only a matter of repetition. Go out on your own a couple of times, and after some weeks you may wonder what the big deal was as you learn that it's fun, that you meet more people, and that it's often easier to get laid as well. Going out on your own has some quite fantastic aspects. One is that you indeed don't know what might happen.

There are adventures to be had out there, and all it takes is a little push. Some guys have told me that they found this step to be surprisingly difficult. If you really think there is a psychological barrier to going out on your own, let alone talking to some random girl, then gradually push your boundaries. Should this apply to you, then your problem isn't night clubs, but social anxiety and feelings of insecurity in general. Maybe it's because you feel exposed. After all, all those people who don't give a fuck about you could secretly be watching you. I'll let you in on a secret: You can experience the same emotions during many activities. Is there some activity you would like to pursue but you keep talking yourself out of it? Just go do it! You will learn that it's quite easy to push your boundaries, and to feel more and more comfortable in your skin.

Doing sports in a group setting, or merely going to the gym may be embarrassing for you. At first you may wonder what all the people think about you, but once you get into working out and show up regularly, the gym starts feeling like home. Eventually your favorite club will feel like that, too. If you want to really put yourself under some pressure, then go to an expensive store after your workout, but in your workout clothes. Shop assistants are normally trained to either get rid of customers who look as if they can't afford the goods on display, or to make them feel very uncomfortable. Keep in mind that you probably make more money than that guy or girl, and that there are no social consequences for having a look at, say, designer furniture in your current outfit. Maybe ask the employees some questions.

Those suggestions may sound a bit inane to you. Yet, if picturing yourself in those situations makes you feel uncomfortable, then think about giving it a shot. If you really want to feel secure about yourself, you could do what I used to do for many years: live modeling. I had been live modeling for fine art students for years, long before I started looking for adventures in all the wrong places. I got into it by accident, but I found that I rather enjoyed striking various poses stark naked in front of an audience mostly consisting of young, attractive women. For me it was a cathartic experience. What's giving a presentation, or going out on your own and trying to bang some random chick compared to that? I don't think you have to go to any extremes, though. No matter what makes you feel uncomfortable, seek out those experiences and learn to deal with them. Desensitizing yourself against social anxiety really is just a matter of practice.

Lastly, if you're afraid that you are going to make a fool out of yourself in your home town, then go to the next bigger city in your area, or deliberately seek out environments where nobody knows you. This should also help you to overcome your inhibitions. However, let me repeat that nobody cares about you. Nobody will keep a close eye on what you are doing. You're effectively invisible to the crowd. Besides, what's the worst that could happen? That some girl you don't know but want to bang asks you why you are going out on your own? You can always say that you just wanted to go out and dance, or listen to music, or be among people. Or you ignore her question. Heck, once I replied to a girl that I just wanted to get laid, while holding eye contact. We left the club together minutes later.

Social pressure

Going out on your own with the aim of pulling girls can be daunting, even if you've had considerable experience with girls. It's not something people normally do. Then again, if you wanted to do what normal people do, you wouldn't have bought this book. Hitting on girls is certainly within the norms of the socially acceptable, as long as you are able to read social cues and don't persist when she is clearly not interested. You can expect to have more success with girls if you go out on your own. But what if you think you just can't do it?

Dealing with social pressure, which is mostly imagined anyway, is something you'll have to learn sooner or later. If you've done some public speaking, you've probably found your first few talks to be fairly intimidating. But as you gained more experience, your nervousness disappeared. You might even have come to enjoy public speaking. It's the same with hitting on girls. You start by making an educated guess. She's looking at you, or brushing her breasts against you as she walks past, so she might be interested on some level. Often, she will then appreciate your initiative if you say hi to her. The first few times you do this, you might find it to be nerve-racking, but eventually, like with public speaking, it won't bother you much anymore.

An objection I've frequently heard is the fear that systematically working on overcoming your inhibitions will make encounters with girls less special. This is not true in general. You will probably care a lot less about some random girl that has the hots for you. With some girls you'll connect on a personal level. However, if you lack sexual experience you only risk reading too much into your interactions with women.

It happens quite often that guys who lack sexual experience end up in relationships that are hardly ideal for them. Being unable to look back on previous relationships or sexual encounters, because there weren't many, or possibly none at all, they can't adequately judge the situation they are in. The guy may not even notice that the girl is only with him because of the promise of financial security, while she sleeps with other guys on the side. Therefore, experience with women will make you realize that many of the encounters you thought were special really weren't, while the rare occurrences where you in fact do connect with someone will be even more remarkable.

Foundations of Success

What do you want?

In life you only ever get what you ask for. As an example, let's consider college applications since most of you are probably familiar with that procedure. Bear with me, because it should soon become clear how all of this relates to picking up girls.

You could be the smartest high school student in the entire United States, but if you don't apply to a place like MIT, you won't ever get in. Applying to a prestigious university brings with it the risk of rejection. To avoid the feeling of rejection, some people choose the safe route. This is reflected in the language of college applications, when students discuss match, stretch, and safety schools. As the wording implies, a safety school is one that, based on your academic record and their admissions statistics, would be very happy to take you. A match school admits people with grades comparable to yours, and the stretch schools are maybe a bit out of reach. Of course, there is a risk that you won't get admitted, but, as I said before, if you don't even apply, then you are guaranteed to not get in anywhere.

In college admissions many students are aware of this distinction. They are advised to maximize their chances by applying to different schools. After all, they want to get in somewhere. Further, you have to make a selection because you can't apply to every university in the world. It's the same when you're looking for a job or when you want to run for a position within an organization.

Dating life is likewise competitive. However, you won't be assessed based on standardized test scores and essays, or your employment history. Instead, what matters most is how you present yourself. Your background, even if there are skeletons in your closet, doesn't matter all that much. This doesn't apply if you've got a city-wide reputation for being a seedy modern Don Juan, but for no-strings-attached sex that's not so bad either. It is startling that many men are very competitive at school or work, yet when it comes to dating they are so desperate that they happily take any woman who wants them.

I'm amazed at the kind of woman some guys settle for. Of course, if both he and she look plain, then they are a good match for each other. However, I can't count the number of men I've seen who were attractive, well-off, or had great earning prospects, and who settled for a woman who looked like a dog. Those women mostly had no redeeming features at all: no proper job, bad education, poorly developed personalities, and no noteworthy interests. Those men were saddling themselves with a liability by pairing up with them. Just like the admissions officers at safety schools, those women were happy to take those guys.

If you go out to a club, looking for a girl to hook up with, I can only advise you to forget about safe bets. Sure, some mediocre looking woman who barely ever gets male attention would be happy to take you, but why on earth would you want to settle for her? You'll be better off going home alone. Really, figure out your market value and only go for girls in the stretch and match category.

This also means that you should forget about hitting on any woman you come across. Some guys refer to this as doing warm-ups, which means that they hit on some girl they don't find attractive, so that they get in the mood of talking to strangers. But this is a horrible idea. It may not always be obvious to her that you are not really interested. In fact, despite the alleged highly developed social skills of women, it is not at all uncommon that they mistake your merely being friendly as romantic interest. She may be happy that any guy talks to her. Yet, it will be obvious to you that you aren't really into her. So what's the point of this then? Certainly you'd much rather have sex with a woman you desire, wouldn't you?

Somewhat related is the problem that the mass media

put a certain image of what is supposed to be attractive in your head. The tall, skinny blonde ranks highly. Yet, not every guy is attracted to this stereotype. Instead, ask yourself whether a particular woman appeals to you. Maybe you like slim brunettes with nice, perky breasts, or maybe you're into redheads who have a big ass. This means that you should also forget about what your friends might think — as long as you are with a girl you really are attracted to, not someone from the bottom of the barrel.

Some guys talk badly about the woman you are about to hook up with, no matter how attractive she is. If she's a skinny blonde he'll call her a bimbo, and if she's a curvaceous brunette he'll remark that he'd rather get with a redhead. He's not hooking up with anybody, but strangely enough he can always find faults with your girls. If you've got a guy like that in your circle of friends, then you might want to consider to stop going out with him.

Go for the kind of woman that turns you on and follow your sexual desire instead of some arbitrary standard of beauty as it is portrayed in movies and advertising. Maybe spend some time thinking about what your goal with pickup is! Do you just want to increase the number of notches on your bedpost or do you want to pursue a particular kind of woman? There are many other possible goals, some of which you may be unaware of.

Maybe you are insecure and want to have sex with a great number of women in order to feel desirable. Of course, wanting to find a great girlfriend is also a viable goal. Whatever your goal may be, make sure that you have some idea of what you want to get out of going to night clubs. If it's really just to hang out with your buddies, then that's fine too, but please don't tell yourself that you only want to hang out with them when you're secretly hoping to meet a nice girl but are afraid to make a move.

Lifestyle choices

As a rule of thumb I would say that if you go out steadily, like two nights a week, you should view yourself as doing pretty okay if you get laid once every month or two. If you are getting laid every other week, then you are doing really great, compared to the average guy. If it's much more often than that, you should be careful because you might burn out on sex and need time to recover. Seduction can take over your life and keep you from getting more worthwhile things done. When I was partying like crazy I had times when I had sex with three different girls just during the week. But please don't ask me what else I have achieved during that time.

A lot of you probably only want to have a nice girlfriend, even if you like to brag about sexual conquests to your buddies. Listen to your desires and don't keep on pulling girls because you enjoy the admiration you get from your male friends. Statements like that normally get feminists fuming, but behold, sisters of Lesbos: The reason why we men admire men who get laid a lot is that it takes conscious effort.

Even if you are a good-looking guy, women will normally not walk up to you, make out, and then drag you back to their place. For this reason we don't even ridicule a guy who occasionally pulls girls who are less than stellar looking. On the other hand, a woman normally only sits or stands there, waiting for guys to show up. It's not much of an exaggeration to say that her part consists of looking good, sending ambiguous signals because she doesn't want to appear to be too easy, and agreeing to get taken home by one of her suitors.

If you secretly only want to have a girlfriend then don't kid yourself and try to pick-up a lot of girls. The women you meet in night clubs may not always be the best candidates for a relationship, but neither will those you meet at work or through your social circle. A lot of women are incredibly screwed-up. I think it's better to go through a lot of women, figure out whether you like them, and let those stick around which you do happen to like. Depending on your spare time or energy you may have to take it slowly. This means that it will take time until you meet someone who might be a suitable partner for you. No, it normally isn't the first woman who is or pretends to be interested in you.

Please take into account that the guys who are doing best with women lead unusual or at the very least rather flexible lives. There is a reason why college students, musicians, artists, or freelancers, guys without real jobs, and entrepreneurs with lifestyle businesses can get more girls, and it has to do with flexibility. Some of the craziest parties I've been to were on Monday nights. Of course, the audience was self-selecting. I don't think I ever met anyone there who had a day job or even just a good reason to get up before 2 p.m. the next day.

Going out from Tuesday to Saturday isn't a viable option if you work 60 hours a week. If this applies to you, then you may want to reconsider your personal goals and think of your long-term happiness. Not all companies work you into the ground. Some are actually quite flexible. A guy I used to hang out with in Berlin had an arrangement with his boss so that he could come to work at 10 or 11 a.m. if there was nothing particularly urgent to do. He didn't have a customer-facing role, did good work, and the company was rather small, so your mileage may vary. Your social life doesn't necessarily have to take a nose dive once you start working. However, I'm well aware that many companies impose artificial deadlines and assign busywork that is essentially pointless.

It's important that you learn to relax and get a clear head. You could play sports, exercise, meditate, take a walk, or countless other things that are not related to your work. A potentially great night will go to waste if you can't get the demanding project you're currently working on, a difficult customer, or office politics out of your mind. Maybe go for a run, and take a nice warm bath before you head to the club.

The pitfalls of being average

You have to find clubs where you feel comfortable, and where you fit in. This probably sounds obvious to you. Yet, judging from the crowd in any club I ever went to, this seems to be obvious to only a small number of people. No matter where you go, most people are just there. It's good that they are there, else the venue would be almost empty. Those people are similar to filler content in consumer products, and not unlike uninspired tracks on albums, unrelated subplots in novels or TV shows, or collectathons and fetch quests in video games. Without those filler people you couldn't run a night, since there is a dearth of cool guys and hot girls. That being said, it's of course possible to rise from those lowly ranks.

Most people are remarkably average. They seem to have no distinctive features, and are overly occupied with fitting in, whatever that may mean in their particular case. Slavishly following fashions, often lagging behind a good year or two, they never develop their own style or even just an original thought of their own. You can notice this with every fad in fashion. When vintage clothing became popular in some circles, those people went out and bought stuff indiscriminately. Or, think of irony as it is celebrated in hipster circles.

Fashion trends are more or less cyclic. What was once mainstream falls out of fashion until it gets picked up again. Rocking a mustache was the thing to do as a male in the '80s, until everybody did it, at which point it became uncool. But lucky you, if you're a hipster, you can grow a mustache and get the admiration of all your mustache-wearing male friends because you don't realize that you're just playing the fashion game on a much smaller scale, following a smaller herd. They also only want to fit in.

You can observe the same behavioral pattern in life in general. Think back to high school for a moment. If your high school was anything like mine, you had three more or less distinct groups. On the bottom of the popularity pole were the geeks, people who were actually interested in something. You know, people who study mathematics in their spare time at a level that goes beyond their textbooks, or teach themselves a programming language. Those are not necessarily the best students, but they most certainly are the smartest.

Others are interested in something other than school. This includes the guy walking around with a copy of Nietzsche's *Thus Spoke Zarathustra*, or the guy who misses half his classes because he wants to spend more time practicing the guitar. Most geeks are not that fortunate and have interests other people tend to find difficult if not impossible to relate to. At the top of the popularity pole are the athletes, the jocks. They look good, are muscular, and they are a hit with the girls. They might not care that much about school otherwise, but why would they, given that they are happy at the moment?

There is also the big fat unremarkable middle, namely

people who don't excel at anything and have no real interests. A few of them may have very good grades, but that's because they have mastered cramming for tests. Ask them some years later to prove the Pythagorean theorem, and they will be stumped. Others want to be popular. They are not as athletic as the jocks, but they suck up to them. They learn how to play the guitar because they think it will help them score with the ladies or they pretend to like certain books or music because they think they are supposed to. Those people are insecure about their status. Bullying normally originates from that group, because in order to cement their position they believe they have to pick on others. Later in life they will almost invariably turn into obnoxious social climbers.

There are advantages to following the beaten path, but the price you pay is your dignity, and any hope to become a mature, confident adult. It may not necessarily be obvious to you yet, but people's life choices are reflected in pretty much everything they do. An average person can't expect non-average results. If you don't know who you are or what you want, then your life will be a collection of random events. Life is not like playing a heavily scripted video game like *Call of Duty* where you follow the lead of some computer-controlled character and always know where you have to go. In real life, blindly following someone's lead can have disastrous consequences that may only become obvious to you years down the line.

Standing out

Disappearing in the crowd is easy. Having a profile is much more difficult, and it may take some time to figure out what you really like. Music is a fitting example since this book is mostly about clubs, but the following applies to any area. Let's talk about a world that might be rather remote from many of you: classical music. I received some years of piano instruction, but never really got anywhere with it. Still, I certainly enjoy listening to classical music. Most classical music performances are safe, though: a Mozart opera, Beethoven's 5th or 9th symphony, or a few piano sonatas by Chopin. I used to work for a promoter of classical concerts, and I can tell you that the repertoire was completely predictable.

The audience those concerts attract are the preposterous middle class, mostly having seemingly no personal taste. Of course, those people were exposed to canonical works of classical music, and have received the message that they are supposed to like it. But did they ever bother to explore the oeuvre of some composer, or try tracing the development of a particular style?

I find it quite amusing that some people maintain a distinction between highbrow and lowbrow culture. Lowbrow is equated with mass culture, having a universal appeal. However, just as, for instance, a video game series like *Call of Duty* appeals to the average gamer who plays whatever he sees advertised on TV, so does the average consumer of classical music only consume what he sees advertised in the media channels he follows. Both are examples of unreflective consumption.

There is a much different world out there, and you only have to look. With a little bit of determination and luck you are bound to discover music, books, or movies you really enjoy. This will go a long way towards developing personal taste. You will probably find that there are certain supposedly great works that are dull. This applies to any area. For instance, virtually every next new great novel will be forgotten within a few years, and only very few works will be held in high regard.

Literature may not be your thing, but the same is true about fashion. There are guys who try to dress like the people in the latest music video of the latest band, but you can likewise take a step back and think for yourself. I like rock music from the '70s, and my clothing style was influenced by it. Skinny black jeans, tight black jacket, black pointy leather shoes, and of course some T-shirts with a band logo. Someone could have worn the same stuff decades earlier and he wouldn't have looked out of place.

Sure, plenty of hipsters probably thought that my clothes weren't edgy or fashionable enough, but I liked them and they conveyed what I wanted to convey. Maybe not everybody feels comfortable looking like a relic from decades past, but if you can pull it off, it will pay off. My style freed me from the pressure of having to update my wardrobe every few months. Further, I can't remember how many times girls tried to start a conversation with me by pointing at my T-shirt, or rubbing it, and saying that they like that band, too.

Polarization

If you have been exposed to the commercial seduction industry, you probably have come across people who claimed that with their system you'll be able to seduce *any* girl. This is a nonsensical claim that is merely supposed to appeal to your delusions of grandeur. What those marketers either implicitly or explicitly say is that one particular method or personal style will get you any girl you want. However, the world is multidimensional. What makes one girl hot and bothered will repel another one.

A better approach to seduction is to become more attractive to a particular group of women. In my seminars I told people to aim to become more attractive to fewer women, which was the main idea of the preceding sections. After all, men who look generic look equally unappealing to all women. Your goal should be to become as attractive as possible to the small subset of women you are actually interested in. This is the idea of polarization brought to its logical conclusion. Why care if 90% of women in the club think you look crazy if 10% really dig your style and a few of those can't wait to spread their legs for you?

Consequently, you should actively seek out venues and activities that enable you to meet the kind of girl you like. For instance, if you are a biker and wanted to pick up some bicker chicks, you'd fix your Harley Davidson and take a ride to the next bar that caters to guys like you. This doesn't mean that every girl will offer to suck your dick the moment you walk in, but by specifically going to places where women who are looking for a guy like you hang out, your odds of getting laid are so much better.

Another important aspect is that seduction is not at all how it is portrayed in the media. There is no Don Juan or Casanova out there who knows a special sequence of words, looks a particular way, or has mannerisms that will eventually and invariably make the woman of his desire give in. This may make for entertaining movies in the best case, but taking those clichés at face value will only lead to frustration in real life.

What happens in reality is that you're seducing women who want to be seduced. They probably weren't looking for you in particular, but for a guy somewhat like you. If you are into blondes and looking for a one-night stand, then probably any decent looking one would do. Women are like us in that regard. For long-term relationships their preferences may shift somewhat, and your earning potential might play a much bigger role, but relationships are hardly the topic of this book.

A lot has been written about so-called game, telling you how to overcome objections, and how to be persistent in the face of resistance. While this may work out in a few cases, it is generally a poor strategy that will make you waste a lot of time. The end result is not particularly appealing either because if you have to force yourself to talk to a woman you don't really feel attracted to, or you trick a girl into bed who doesn't fancy you all that much, then the outcome can't be that pleasurable. In the worst case you end up with a woman who only uses you for validation, doesn't make a particular effort to please you in bed, might even treat you badly, and who you aren't really horny for, either. The more game you need to get her, the worse the result will be.

Getting the Edge

Looking the part

On my forum some guy once wrote, "But how do you pull that stuff off if you lack those foundations, i.e. what kind of advice can you give for people with an average fashion sense and an average physical appearance?" This may sound like a valid objection, and it's not an uncommon one. Among guys who don't have much success with girls at all, or who happen to get lucky every once in a while, there often is the attitude that they were dealt a certain hand in life, and that's all there is to it. The mere suggestion that they should get in shape makes them react defensively. Apparently they think that it's shallow to work out, but on the other hand it's not shallow at all if you're a lazy guy and entertain fantasies about boning some girl who happens to be in shape. She goes to the gym to look good, so shouldn't you work out, too?

Some people drastically underestimate how much they

can change. Your haircut doesn't have to be boring, and, with the exception of some exceedingly rare medical issues, obesity can be fought as well. You can change if you want! All it takes is dedication and enough time. By the way, I wasn't exactly a sporty kid. It would have been a bit of a stretch to refer to my sixteen-year-old self as fat, but I certainly was on the pudgy side, partly due to my mother's fondness for baking cakes, often one or two per week. She also used to buy my clothes. Frankly, I didn't care all that much about clothes, so it didn't bother me that much, which is an attitude I kept for a long time. I don't write this to get your sympathy but to illustrate that my starting position was not ideal either.

If you never spent time thinking about fashion, or the absurdity of ever-changing fashions, then you may believe that some people know something about this topic which you don't. However, there is no fashion gene. All it takes is the will to experiment, and a bit of spare change. With a bit of ingenuity you won't wreck your finances either.

There are other resources that tell you about getting into shape. There aren't so many that teach you how to develop a sense for fashion, so the remainder of this chapter will be on that topic. You should not think that this is superfluous. Assuming you are in reasonable shape, meaning at the very least toned, your success hinges a lot on how you present yourself. In the hectic club environment, which allows for quick hookups, even deficiencies in your personality don't count for much. They will, should you want to get into a relationship, but if you want to have one-night stands, you basically just need to be there, have a somewhat distinct look, find a girl who is interested, and move the interaction forward.

A lesson from women

Helena Rubinstein, founder of the eponymous chain of beauty products and salons famously said, "There are no ugly women, only lazy ones." You have to consider that beauty was her business and that she was, quite successfully, playing into the insecurities of women in order to make money. When she died, she was one of the wealthiest women in the United States. Her brand still lives on.

Advertising rhetoric aside, there is a lot of truth in Rubinstein's dictum. Of course, there are some issues you can't fix without plastic surgery, and some where not even that would help much. But take your regular plain Jane: she doesn't work out, doesn't care much about what she eats, and doesn't put much thought into clothes and make-up. Obviously, she will at best be mildly attractive. Even worse, if she lives in a culture in which she suffers no social consequences for looking unattractive, she probably won't change a thing.

I've been told that in some Asian countries there is societal pressure on women to be slim, and if they start to gain even just a little bit of weight, her female friends and family, especially her mother, will mock her relentlessly. Now compare this to a culture of complacency like the United States or most European countries where it isn't rare that good-looking women who make a conscious effort to look their best are sometimes chided for looking like hookers or wannabe porn stars. You would be surprised if you knew how nasty girls are towards each other. Since one girl trying to look better would make her peers look worse, she has to be kept in check. It would be the opposite if, say in a group of female volleyball players, one of the girls would gain weight.

But back to plain Jane! Imagine she began working out and shedding those pounds. Then she could let her hair grow, and learn to apply make-up to make her more appealing. Once she gets new clothes, she'll (almost) be a bombshell. There are plenty of men who can look past, for instance, a big nose or a flat chest, if the girl has amazing thighs and a firm ass. Preferences obviously differ, and while there are some guys who are fat fetishists and refer to the objects of their desires as big beautiful women, the majority of men prefers having a healthy-looking mate.

What men can do

A woman can make herself look relatively attractive with a little bit of effort. Many don't do that, instead preferring to complain that there are no good men around anymore, whatever that might mean. As a guy you can likewise complain that the women are too picky or that you only get laid rather randomly. But are you sure you have maximized your looks? If you think you are ugly or unattractive, then get a sticky note and write down: "I can look good." Put it on your fridge so that you will constantly be reminded of it.

I'm not going to delve into self-help mumbo jumbo, but merely want you to consider how you can improve your looks. What's even better is that there is not only a wider variety of what constitutes sexy men, looks are also less important than with women. A woman may not get a second glance if she isn't appealing enough. Yet, if you are a guy, many women will cut you some slack.

She has to be somewhat attracted to you, obviously, but she'll judge everything you bring to the table, especially for longer relationships. Your status counts, your education may count, your job certainly does, and also your bank account. For one-night stands looks are much more important than your wallet if she really only wants to have sex and nothing else, but you'll find that many women at first give the impression that they are only interested in some kind of casual arrangement, before they suddenly get clingy.

Being unattractive is for the very most part a choice. It is a choice many people make without being aware of it. If you are not getting anywhere with women, start with the very foundations. Lose some weight, fix your hygiene, and look as good as you possibly can. Bigger muscles don't necessarily mean that you'll get laid more often, but you'll at least appeal to a very specific group of women. In any case, women want a guy who looks healthy, and for this reason it's better to be slender than fat. Long gone are the times where a big belly was a status symbol.

Lastly, I have to point out that you can even turn what you may consider weaknesses into strengths on the dating market. It may sound odd to you, but some women dig guys who look like thugs, or at least dangerous. One of my friends got into a bad accident once, and as a reminder he now has a big scar on his left arm. However, once a girl he was with told him that it turned her on, he began flaunting it. He thought he had to hide it, but as he found out, it can be an asset.

A different take on fashion

In my not so humble opinion, fashion is a scam of enormous proportions. The fashion industry tells you every three months that it's time to get some new clothes so that you can keep fitting in. However, once you go out and buy some stuff, it won't take that long until there are some new colors that are all the rage, or different styles that are either invented or rejuvenated. The fashion industry holds out a carrot, and the general public rushes out to get some new clothes, not realizing that while they are pulling out their credit cards to pay for a new set of trendy clothes, the next two to three trends have already been designed by the various labels.

There is a different way to tackle the problem of how to look appealing without degrading yourself. The key is following certain stereotypes. Over the last few decades a number of styles have turned out to have tremendous lasting appeal. Taking some cues from the history of rock music, I got myself pointy leather shoes, tight black jeans, flashy T-shirts, and dark blazers. Taken out of context, I could have been a Rolling Stones fan from the 1960s. Likewise, picture a biker with his leather gear, sitting on his Harley Davidson! Out of context you might have a hard time guessing which decade he is from.

If you compare the lasting appeal of those stereotypes with today's fashion, you'll probably notice that the latter is a sucker's bet. Jeans change from blue to black, from skinny to baggy, from capri to too long, and from pressed to vintage within a few years. However, the old pair of Levi's 501 a biker wears when he's checking the brakes of his motorcycle has remained unchanged for at least a few decades. Indeed, one benefit of picking a stereotype is that you won't have to spend much time or money updating your wardrobe. It will probably take you a while to find some decent clothes in the beginning, and fitting accessories. However, afterwards you could easily choose to only replace your clothes once they are worn out.

No matter what kind of stereotype you're going to go for, even if it is *Jersey Shore* douchebag style, there are some constants. First, you should make sure that the clothes fit your body. If you want to strut around in tight jeans in an indie rock bar, you better not have much fat, or muscle, on your bones. The edgier styles are sometimes difficult to pull off. Indeed, it's a fine line between looking cool and looking like a travesty. For tight clothes you have to be in the right shape.

Body fit doesn't necessarily mean that everything has to be tight. Instead, your clothes should look good on you. Normally you would want to avoid wearing clothes that are too big. A mistake I commonly see is guys who are a bit overweight wearing baggy clothes, which only makes them look even more out of shape. You'll look a lot better in clothes you don't disappear in.

On that note, you may need to take up sports or start lifting weights. A little bit of muscle makes an enormous difference. It will improve your health, and it will make you more attractive to women. Speaking about myself as a guy who roamed an environment in which every other guy was wearing skinny jeans and pointy shoes as well: by having a bit of muscle, toned rather than bulked up, I stood out of the crowd, since most of those guys were so slim that they looked downright unhealthy.

By going for certain stereotypes you polarize. Well, in some environments it's your only way to get in anyway. With a bit more effort you will also notice that a lot more women notice you. They spend easily an hour or more on their appearance before going out, and if you take an extra ten or fifteen minutes to fix your clothes you'll probably be ahead of most other guys.

Of course stereotyping to some extent means taking on

44

a different role. We aren't all tough bikers or wannabe rockstars, and the girls you're going to meet aren't high-society queens, or lead-singers in a band either. But there is some appeal to being more than your boring regular self for a few hours, once or twice a week.

What girls look for

In *Club Game* I don't assume that you've been exposed to game as it is promoted by so-called pickup artists (PUAs). There are many ways to critique their methods, and I've done so in some of my other works. Let me therefore briefly draw your attention to one of their biggest falla-cies. If you are familiar with some of the bigger names in this scene, you've surely seen guys wearing furry hats and boots with ten-inch soles, or people with a multi-colored Iroquois haircut. No matter how bizarre, there is probably a PUA out there who endorses that kind of garishness.

What those people fail to grasp is that women do not look for such caricatures. PUAs are not part of popu-lar culture, and women certainly haven't grown up with a positive image of them. The media exposure they sometimes get is due to the novelty factor they provide. On the other hand, girls grow up marveling at musi-cians, athletes, and actors. No matter who she is, there most certainly are some famous men whose look she has grown to like.

In fact, no matter where you go, women will look for their kind of guy. This is most visible in any kind of sub-culture. There are emos, rockers, punks, skaters, goths, and whatnot. If she styled herself to be an emo girl, then she is going to be much more interested in hooking up with a guy who shares her fashion orientation. In fact, in non-mainstream clubs the look of the audience is shaped by the style of the bands and musicians they idolize. This is not so different from some girl who goes to work in high heels and a costume who'd much prefer a guy in a suit over some sleaze who pretends to play in a band.

Today's and yesterday's music heroes didn't operate in a vacuum, however, and have taken cues from their pre-decessors. Those were refined, but with some effort you could construct a fashion timeline, highlighting influ-ences from, say, the Rolling Stones to The Kooks, or from The Talking Heads to Panic at the Disco. Don't worry about those bands if you don't recognize them. Feel free to look up images of them online, but rest as-sured that they will be forgotten sooner or later anyway. Names and faces change, but underlying styles don't. There will always be bands whose members dress in a very eccentric style, and others who prefer some under-statement.

To give you a concrete example, let me point out that the classic rockstar stereotype has evolved since the days of Iggy Pop and Ozzie Osbourne. But 2000's Iggy doesn't look too different from the 1970's. Similarly, a more con-temporary band like The Horrors shows the influence of the style of The Rolling Stones, but their stylists went to some extremes, working on haircuts and make-up you probably could only pull off in very few clubs, provided you had make-up artists and hair stylists at hand to fix your look.

Traditional fashion resources

For an education on the basics of fashion you might want to have a look at textbooks on fashion design. I once skimmed a few books to great effect at my local library. Given the inflated prices of textbooks, and the limited use you'll get from such a book, I wouldn't recommend buying any of those, though. To put things into comparison: for the price of such a textbook I had gotten a complete basic outfit for my "Sleazy Rockstar" persona and money left over for accessories.

Some sources are better skimmed, like books on certain designers. Those usually make for great coffee table books, and may make a nice addition to your personal library, if you are into collecting books. Look up a few well-known male designers, and see whether there are books showcasing their creations. Pay attention to how they subtly change themes, and with which colors they work. Check your local library first before you splurge on those books, though, since, again, these won't be books you'll be spending a lot of time with.

Glossy magazines for men, like GQ, or women's magazines like Elle or Cosmopolitan are little more than ads for luxury labels. At best I would have a look at them to get an idea for how to combine certain colors, or get an idea on current styles, if you want to take some cues on that. In general, though, I would stay away from them, not just because they highlight office or street wear. You will certainly look nice if you follow their advice. It probably won't give you an edge, but it might bleed your bank account dry. If you are stuck at an airport, or waiting for a train and you've got ten minutes to spare, then go to a newsstand and skim a few magazines. Doing this somewhat regularly for a few weeks should be sufficient to get a feel for colors and fit.

Contemporary fashion resources

There are plenty of blogs run by people who specialize in either street fashion, document the styles that are popular in particular night clubs, or possibly even cover entire scenes. This may help, but the quality is rather uneven. Had I not known what to look for, those sources would have confused rather than helped me. Keep this option in the back of your mind, but don't use it yet. You may find that you'll be fine without.

If you know some bands whose music you like, and if it's music that is being played in the clubs you like going to, then it can't hurt to check the websites of those bands for inspiration. Many of the more fashion-concerned patrons in trendy clubs do the same. While you may find it hard to copy the outfit of musicians, you'll certainly get a few good ideas here and there. The reason why you often won't be able to copy their outfit is because the more outlandish pieces were designed specifically for them. Of course, if you've got the money, I don't want to discourage you from spending a few grand on a bespoke leather jacket.

Should you happen to live in a bigger city with a visible gay scene you should check out some of their clubs. You will probably meet a few rather open-minded girls in those clubs, too, but an added benefit is that gay men tend to be on the forefront of fashion. This environment might make you feel uncomfortable, but keep in mind that gay men tend to be open-minded, and not obtrusive at all. It's not the case that they would hit on you the way some guys hit on girls.

Gay men just talk to you, and may offer you sex almost as nonchalantly as you would ask a friend whether he'd like to have a beer. But if you don't agree to it, they'll accept that, and if they like you, they may keep talking to you for a bit nonetheless. In gay scenes sex is no big deal. I had the impression that gay men spend very little time on courting, and that people mainly socialize. Sex happens so quickly in that scene that it seems to only be an added benefit.

All of this might change once gay culture becomes part of the mainstream, but for the time being you can get plenty of good ideas about fashion from gay men. Indeed, many styles that became popular in cities like London and New York, before they spread over the globe, emerged in gay clubs first. This was true for skinny jeans before the mainstream picked them up, or for checkered shirts, which were popular in the gay scene years before you could buy them in regular stores.

Whom not to listen to

As a precautionary note I'll add that there are two common sources you should not listen to. Well, the third one would be your mother. In general, it doesn't serve you well to listen to the advice girlfriends and female friends give. For one, women normally don't have much of a clue about fashion and tend to follow trends without thinking much about it. They certainly don't know what suits men, and for their own clothes they stick very close to the images presented to them in stores and women's magazines.

If you've had a couple of non-serious relationships, you may be tempted to ask your lovers for advice. In this case, the problem is that she may want to reel you into a serious relationship and start by turning you into a nice guy, clothes-wise. After all, what interest could she possibly have to make you look more attractive to other women? She's probably glad to have you in her life. Asking her for assistance to improve your chances with her rivals is therefore downright absurd.

I would also stay away from the advice of shopping assistants. I don't want to claim that they are all bad, but if you don't know what looks good on you, you would have to take their advice at face value. They primarily want to sell you something — anything —, and if you look clueless, they might try to sell you the most over-priced and least in-demand items they can find. Let me tell you an anecdote from my time in Berlin, when I was going through a phase where I was collecting neckties. I was actually the only guy in the office wearing them. Then again, a touch of dandyism isn't something I view as negative. Looking for bargains I went to an upscale haberdasher in one of the more upscale areas in Berlin. I should add that my regular outfit during the day consists of sneakers, T-shirt, skinny jeans, and, if it's not warm enough, a hoodie.

Visualizing my outfit you probably can't blame the shop assistant for thinking that there's another sucker coming in. My first question was whether they had any neckties for sale. Fine silk neckties from Milan would normally have been too much for my budget, so I was willing to take a gamble and have a look at last season's collection. For more classical patterns the fashion hardly changes anyway. The shop assistant showed me the way and as we arrived at that section of the store, she started bull-shitting me and recommended a handful of neckties. I told her that I was fine on my own, and dug out a number of great neckties, all at a fraction of their regular price. The stuff she wanted to sell would neither have looked good, nor was the quality particularly impressive, and she indeed looked surprised when I went to the till with those carefully selected pieces and, yes, got some excellent Italian silk ties for a pretty good price that afternoon.

Before we move on to the next part, let me add that if you think that all of this sounds like a lot of effort, then consider what women go through. The bar for men is pretty low. When I was living in Berlin, I got the impression that you already stood out from the crowd already if you wore fitting clothes and washed your face. People in London pay much more attention to fashion, but it's still nothing compared to the effort women make. There are literally hundreds of shades of red lipstick, and chances are that she'll choose one to match the tone of her new red dress. In a double-blind test those women probably wouldn't be able to tell the difference between various shades of red, so this entire charade is quite comical. Yet, lipstick is only the beginning. Many women spend countless hours putting together their outfits.

Party

Club Sociology

Clubs and social circles

Meeting girls through one's wider social circle, particularly for more serious relationships, works quite well. In fact, it is by far most common to meet a partner in school or at the workplace. However, depending on where you are in your life, night clubs and bars may be an infinitely better resource, particularly if you are primarily interested in sexual gratification. Unlike your social circle, in a club you can meet dozens of interesting women night after night, and that's out of the hundreds that go there. Even if you had access to a very large social circle, you'd probably find it quite difficult to encounter more than half a dozen fresh faces a month.

A big downside of social circles is that it takes a long time to build one. Once you are out of college you may find that your days basically consist of working, sleeping and running errands. Calling random acquaintances and fostering friendships will thus probably be lower on your list of priorities. Further, it takes quite an effort to maintain a social circle, if you are at all concerned about having non-superficial friendships. In college it's easy to hang out with your buddies, but once that's over, keeping in touch with more than your closest friends becomes a real challenge.

Instead of growing your social circle, you could maintain friendships with the guys you know. This is a common strategy, and it will mean that many of those people will eventually disappear from your life. People move away, marry, or develop different interests. For the purpose of picking up girls, hanging out with a more or less fixed group of people can be counterproductive. Indeed, many decisions will be based on the lowest common denominator. Before you know it you all sit in a movie nobody actually wanted to watch, but all thought would be a good compromise.

I don't oppose the idea of having friends or meeting people for the sake of socializing. However, if your aim is to get laid, then the pay-off is quite bad. Just compare the incredible amount of time you have to invest in your social circle with the actual results! On the other hand, anyone who has found a few clubs he really enjoys going to can get laid with so much less effort, and with a much higher number of women, that it puts all but the most popular socializers to shame.

I haven't even covered the issue of rank within groups. Active social circles tend to grow over time, and they are normally bound to a particular city or, at best, a relatively narrow geographic area. This means that if you move to a new city you won't be able to take your old social circle with you. Instead, you'll have to start over once again. Having a few contacts, possibly old friends, will give you a head start. Still, you won't be the leader of that social circle, and you won't decide where to go or what to do. This will probably suck for quite some time. Eventually new people join, allowing you to slowly move up in the ranks. By the way, the guy at the top of the pyramid can't just ditch the group because he wants to chase after some girls. He'll have obligations to the group as well.

Social circle game has further drawbacks for guys with demanding jobs. Your spare time is limited, and you'll often find that you'd rather relax in the evening or re-cover on the weekend. This is especially the case if you don't get enough sleep during the week. If you have to travel a lot due to work, you'll probably never fully es-tablish yourself in your city. By the time you've gotten to know some people the guys you've met two years ago are about to get married or leave the city again. In short, you'll never leave square one as all your private contacts are of a rather fleeting nature.

It doesn't end there, though. I have spent many years in big cities like London or Berlin, and even though I had plenty of spare time, I quickly learnt that it's not that easy to build a social circle. Sure, you'll meet a lot of people, but your contacts will normally be rather super-ficial, meaning that you'll find yourself socializing with people you interact with anyway, either through your job or studies, or some sport you pursue.

For the sexual deviants among you, I'll lastly draw attention to the fact that social circles normally won't give you much room for experimentation. Once people know you, they expect you to play a certain role, but as you know, one's personality is multi-faceted. Your work colleagues see a different you than your old buddies from high school. Especially when you feel like testing out your sexuality or trying to play a different role at night, you may find that your social circle limits you. The women you're going to meet will primarily ask themselves whether you are boyfriend material. All of this is bad news if you bought a bag of sex toys last weekend and wanted to find out whether it is really true that girls on one-night stands are more experimental than those you had to date for weeks before you got to second base.

On a related note, relying too much on your social circle to meet women can easily make you complacent and give you a false sense of security. I often witness guys attempting to get with a girl in their wider social circle, not realizing that they have no chance at all. Mistaking her friendliness as a sign of interest, those guys then expend a tremendous amount of energy. In a different setting, like in a club or bar, they wouldn't have deluded themselves to believe that they are slowly making progress.

What's good about social circles

Social circle game can work if you set yourself up so that you can hop *between* several groups. Instead of aiming to strengthen your position within one particular group, you are the guy many people kind of know. Everybody is happy to see you because you are an interesting character. If they knew you better, you would appear to be more bland, but probably anybody can be a fun guy for twenty minutes. Furthermore, everyone will be happy to see you because they know that you'll soon be gone anyway. I don't intend this to be a cynical remark. Sure, some people you know will genuinely like you, but many are phonies who pretend to like everyone, and a phony will find it much easier to pretend to like you if she only bumps into you every few weeks, and you chat a bit with some people in her group before you head off again.

A consequence of the strategy I just outlined is that people will cut you quite some slack. You surely have met guys like this. It's the seemingly outgoing character that shakes your hand, maybe gives you a quick hug, exchanges a few words with you to update you on his life, and gives you the chance to do the same. People probably don't miss him much, but he's a nice addition, and he brings some life into the gatherings of maybe somewhat boring dudes sitting for far too long in a bar or pub after work on a Friday evening. Heck, maybe nobody knows what that guy is really doing or how it happened that he knew them, but he shows up every now and then, is friendly, and provides some distraction.

The latter was certainly a role I enjoyed playing. There were quite a few people in Berlin or London I knew I would bump into, and when I saw them I had a quick chat with them. There were some whose name I never remembered, and of whom I neither knew where they lived or how I could reach them. Of some I had contact details but rarely got in touch with them. If at all, it was to coordinate plans every once in a while. Making deep connections wasn't the point anyway. Still, if you hang out in a place you like, and you see a friendly face you know, you probably wouldn't mind having a quick chat with him. Basically nobody is opposed to talking to someone for while. This includes girls, particularly if it is clear that you do not intend to hit on them.

Hopping between social circles and maintaining loose connections leads to club game. Think of a club as a very large social circle with rather limited interpersonal bonds. Yes, they are all friends, but not quite like friends. They are all friendly towards each other, and they all like hanging out in that place or go out in that scene. The big group is more important than the individual in those settings, and in a way they are all hopping from one loose social circle, i.e. club, to another within their scene. This is why, if you happen to find a scene you really enjoy, you will bump into many people over and over.

If you play your cards right, club game can give you all the benefits of social circles, and much more! Club game will also spare you the crap you have to deal with in social circles. Let's be honest here: How much do you really care about all the people you frequently hang out with? Probably not all that much. There are maybe one or two people you like a lot, your close friends, and the others are often just there. My social life in London and Berlin was a consequence of those insights. I had a few close friends, but when I wanted to get my rocks off I went to clubs, and frequently on my own. I knew I'd know some faces there, and that there would be no shortage of girls to meet.

Understanding clubs

If you aren't familiar with night clubs you may very well think that they are all the same. Probably images of the kind of clubs the *Jersey Shore* cast appeared in come to mind. However, while mainstream clubs that play the Top 40 up and down are all rather similar, differences between clubs are actually quite substantial.

A big factor is obviously the music they play. Compared to an indie rock venue, a techno club has a much different feel to it, and therefore there normally aren't that many people who would feel equally at home in both scenes. It is often the case that clubs that cater to people who are interested in a certain kind of music don't have a rigid door policy. They want everyone who likes the music they play to come and spend some money. Sometimes the doormen will point out that the music may not be to your taste. When I was about to check out an R'n'B club in Berlin the guy at the door said to me, in a friendly tone, that I was very welcome to come in, but that I should know that their audience was primarily teenagers, and that they only played black music.

There are also clubs that target certain age groups. For instance, in Germany it's legal to enter clubs from age 16 onward. The law states that if you are under 18 you have to leave by midnight, but this normally doesn't deter high school students from using a fake ID. As a consequence, some clubs draw the line at 21 or even 25. Even if there is no 21+ sign, the doormen might nonetheless be instructed to send away anybody who looks too young. At the other end of the spectrum you'll find scenes that are often frequented by people who are a bit older. I've been to quite a few techno clubs where most were in their late twenties. Further, in the swinger scene it's said to be rare to find someone under 30. I hopefully do not have to point out that you should try to find places where you fit in. In any larger city this shouldn't be overly difficult.

It can't hurt to think about the district the club is located in. Larger cities normally have tourist districts where the beer is pricey, the food bad, and the service substandard. Clubs in those districts tend to aim for the lowest common denominator. Whether this is good or bad is up to you to decide. If you want to try your luck with some ladies from abroad, it may be a good choice. But if you have more than a one-night stand in mind you better find clubs that are frequented by the locals as well.

The next way to categorize clubs is all too obvious to guys who go out frequently, but people who regularly stay in are often completely unaware of it. I'm talking about underground clubs as opposed to mainstream clubs. Mainstream clubs are the previously mentioned clubs for the lowest common denominator. Everybody wearing a white shirt and blue jeans gets in, it seems, and no matter which day you go there, they play the same 20 tracks over and over. Everything is loud. Every cab driver knows where they are, and they advertise a lot.

On the other hand, underground clubs often survive on word of mouth. Some are illegal, meaning that the owner doesn't have a license to sell alcohol. Those may be recurring events, or one-time-only parties in some abandoned warehouse. To limit access for the uninitiated, they may send out passwords to people via text messages or email. All those antics may look childish to you, but if you've been to those events, you know that they can be rather special since they are a bit smaller, and have an incredibly open atmosphere. Even if they suck, they suck in a more interesting way than your standard mainstream venue.

You could make many more distinctions, but the ones I just mentioned I consider to be the main differentiators. In any case, I hope you got the point that every club is different, not just because they cater to a certain crowd or play a particular kind of music. You should therefore make a deliberate choice about where to go out to and don't do what many guys seem to do, which is going out randomly. They try two or three clubs, until they get in somewhere. However, with some preparation their nights could go so much better.

The doorman

There is nothing preventing you from hitting on girls in the queue to the club, but you'll probably agree that the night starts once you're inside, no pun intended. But before that, you'll have to find the approval of the guys at the door. In mainstream clubs it's primarily a matter of wearing clean clothes and not showing up too late, because they keep a close eye on the male-to-female ratio. It's not that other clubs don't care about that ratio, apart from places that gather to a primarily homosexual clientele. Rather, the way you style yourself is of utmost importance. Some clubs even gain notoriety for their allegedly tough door policy, such as Berghain in Berlin.

The doorman decides who gets in. If he doesn't like you, you can try your luck somewhere else. At more mainstream clubs you sometimes see guys walk all the way to the front of the queue, shaking the hand of the bouncer, and getting welcomed in. This is normally bribery. Just fold up a 50 or 100 dollar bill, stick it between your pinkie and ring finger, and — important! — tilt your hand slightly outward as you stretch out your hand so that the bouncer knows what's coming up.

On the other hand, in subcultures money doesn't help all that much. Instead, you have to know about the dress code of that scene, and if you do, you won't have to fear the doorman. To people not in the know the selection process in the queue seems random. To them it feels as if they are at that guy's mercy, but I could fairly reliably predict if the people in front of me would get in or not. Some people look so out of place that they would get turned away even if the club was empty.

Plain and simple, the guy at the door plays an important role in determining the fate of the club. The patrons rely on the club bringing together people that are like them, so that no one is put out of their comfort zone, but instead gets their ego stroked due to the affirmation they directly or indirectly receive from all the others who dress like them. I don't want to sound cynical though, because it is great to go to a club the very first time and feel right at home, have a fabulous time with random people, make some new friends you'll have forgotten about the next day, and take some girl home.

Club promoters of off-beat nights seem aware of the desire of their patrons to belong, in some fuzzy sense, and therefore they put great emphasis on their door policy. In mainstream clubs on the other hand, people are apparently hell-bent on milking a club night for as long as possible, before changing its name and interior, and this is what I consider cynical. If the bouncer selects people who don't chime with each other, everybody will feel uncomfortable, and plenty of people won't come back.

Maybe you've experienced a big group coming into a club, projecting a rather negative vibe that ruins the atmosphere of the entire place. It doesn't have to be a stag or hen party, although that is an extreme example of that phenomenon. After enough bad nights, whatever your personal limit is, you probably won't come back anytime soon. In big cities there are enough clubs you could carry your money to, so competition for the in-crowd is intense. Consequently, a bad door policy can wreck a once successful club night within a few months.

Let's assume it's a well-run club, and that they put on some really great nights. You want to get in, but you are unsure of yourself. Thankfully, the selection criteria are rather objective, for all the reasons I just mentioned. The doorman will look at your clothes, and your stance. If you look insecure or as if you don't belong he may quickly send you on your way again, even if there is nothing wrong with your clothes. As long as you look as if you fit into that place and you're not too wasted, you shouldn't have any problems. There are plenty of scenes where it's better to look a bit fucked-up, though. However, make sure you don't look like trouble, i.e. don't be loud or aggressive. Especially younger guys seem to think that making a bad impression is a good idea.

You might be concerned about your age, especially if you're past 25. Don't worry too much about it. In non-mainstream clubs age is much less of an issue. When I was going out in the techno scene in Berlin most people were in their mid to late twenties. Sometimes you'd bump into teenagers, and you could just as well end up talking to a guy in his fifties. The older men wouldn't wear sneakers and a bright tight shirt, but with a nice suit or good jeans and expensive shoes they wouldn't make a fool of themselves on the dance floor either. Seeing a woman in her late 30s is a rare sight in those places, though — or maybe I simply never noticed them. After all, guys have got a good extra ten years of youth compared to women, and if you play your cards right, you can easily get women ten years younger than you.

But what if the doorman tells you that you're not getting in? In that case you should not feel bad about yourself. In fact, he just did you a great favor. It's good that you were turned away because you wouldn't have fit in anyway! The girls would have ignored you, and the guys as well. In some environments the people would have made fun of you. Let me tell you about one of my favorite clubs back in London. They had an absolutely fabulous night every Wednesday, and the crowd was, well, not quite what I would call normal. People were doing coke in the open, and sex in a bathroom stall was a frequent occurrence.

While a girl was massaging your cock in your pants as she was talking to you, it could happen that someone slid up to you, stuck his pinkie under your nose and told you have some.[1] I thought it was a place of magic and

---

[1] If this does not make sense to you: Among people who take cocaine regularly and like to celebrate this fact, it is common to let the the nail of the pinkie of your dominant hand grow a bit longer, so that it is easier to shuffle cocaine with it. No, I don't think this is very hygienic, but I'd say that having a coke habit in the first place is more worrisome.

67

wonder, and I rarely felt happier among people, since they weren't judgmental in any way. Well, that was if you got in. However, sometimes, you would see a couple of regular guys in there as well, maybe more for the entertainment of the staff than the patrons. It was quite an odd sight to see two poorly dressed frightened pale guys, with a confused look on their face, standing next to half naked men who were getting hot and heavy with each other. I bet those poor souls wished to have been refused entry.

If you can't seem to figure out how to get into a particular club despite your best efforts, you can try showing up early as a last-ditch effort. This is often pointless in more popular clubs because they can afford to send people away. There are probably limits to your willingness to change yourself to get into a certain place, so at one point you'll probably be better off by moving on.

When it comes to more mainstream clubs it's common that guys, no matter how good-looking or well-off, have to bring an equal number of girls with them to get in. In that case you can either bribe the doorman, or bring some girls with you next time. But, honestly, I never understood why you would want to go out with a girl, assuming you fuck her. Well, if those clubs are so important to you and you don't know any girls, then arrive earlier next time, or don't go again. Apparently they think you don't fit, or are too old, or too young, or whatever else. Or maybe you don't look as if you would spend a lot of money in there.

Not having girls with you is sometimes only a pretense to refuse entry, though, and it wouldn't really help you to bring girls with you. I've even seen guys in the company of pretty hot girls get sent away, like at Berghain in Berlin. The reason was of course that they would not have fit in. I probably don't have to mention this, but comments like "today, guest list only" or "this place is only for regulars" all mean that they don't want to have you in there, and you should be glad they let you know. Better go to a place where you can meet girls who look for a guy like you, instead of trying to get into a club where you'd stick out like a sore thumb.

Picking the right clubs

Probably in every city there are a few clubs or bars that have a reputation for being chock-full of easy girls. This is mostly nonsense. If Joe Average gets shot down in some club by a random girl, he'll go around telling others that it's impossible to get laid there. On the other hand, should he get lucky in some other venue, or a friend of his, it's suddenly an easy place to get laid.

If it's a venue you like, and a scene you fit in, you'll find that it doesn't matter so much where you go since your chances of getting laid are more or less the same. Therefore, I would suggest you forget about choosing clubs based on your belief of where it's easiest to get laid. Instead, take it as a given that if it's the right kind of club for you, you'll have a realistic chance to get laid. After all, girls go to clubs precisely for that reason, and if she's claiming the opposite, she's probably lying. A girl who is not interested in meeting men, or one who is in a relationship, has no business going to a club and complaining when men hit on her. She is wearing high heels, a tight skirt, and a push-up bra, after all. Thus, she is looking, even if only subconsciously.

Primarily, make sure it's a club you like, and the rest will follow. I can't stress this point enough. Even if you end up in a scene where there are many more men around, if it's an environment you truly enjoy, it will be obvious to other people. They will like you for that, and girls will notice it as well. You can even get laid as a straight guy on a gay and lesbian club night, provided you manage to get in.

In a small city you normally don't have much choice, but if you happen to live in or near a metropolis, then please do make an effort and do some research. First, narrow down the list according to music. If you like the music, and dress accordingly, then half the battle is won already since you won't hate yourself for singing along to whatever the music industry recently churned out, but instead bop your head to music you like, and might even listen to at home.

If this leaves too many venues on your list, then you can view yourself as being in a very fortunate position. You can now go to the places with the atmosphere you like best. Chances are that if you are having a blast, and like the people, you will find it very easy to get laid. A different approach is to pick a place that makes it easier to get laid. Berghain in Berlin is infamous for that, where the layout of the club encourages people to have sex inside the venue. Alternatively, pick a club that is reasonably close to your apartment, or easy to get to via public transport.

Going out with friends

I recommend going out on your own. Alternatively, go out with one or two male friends, but only if two conditions are met: they are able to talk to women by themselves, and they actually do it. I have often experienced that guys I went out with tried to take over the conversation when I was talking to a girl, which I found to be rather irritating.

Even worse, when confronted, their responses ranged from denying that they were messing up my interactions to accusing me of being selfish for wanting to have some girl for myself. Some guys even asked me incredulously why I was complaining, since I was so good with girls anyway. However, I also meet guys who were pretty much like me. We would either go to the club together, or arrange to meet inside, but the latter didn't always work out so well because it happened quite frequently that one of us had already left with some girl before we were able to catch up.

If you are able to find guys like that, then I can only encourage you to go out with them. On the other hand, if your male friends are like most guys I met, you may as well go out on your own. I've already mentioned that your wingman can easily end up ruining the early phase of an interaction with a girl, but the problem runs deeper. Most guys are simply another person to take care of.

Some guys may even complain if you walk off to hit on a girl, and then there are of course those who only go to clubs to drink and want you to stay with them at the bar so that they don't have to feel like losers for drinking alone. But please don't get me wrong! I'm not at all against hanging out with people. However, if you want to pull some girls, you probably shouldn't socialize with the most insecure guys you know.

I consider going out with groups to be a bad idea in general. Everybody's got an opinion about which club they would like to go to, but if you suggest one of the trendier places in your city, there will always be someone who complains. Maybe it's because they never got in. Plenty of the more interesting places have a relatively restrictive door policy, and some won't let groups in at all since too many groups ruin the atmosphere. I had a particularly noteworthy encounter once in Berlin, when I met some guys for drinks, non-alcoholic ones in my case, in the evening in one of the bars in the Kreuzberg district.

It was a lively place, and the group at our table got bigger and bigger. Two hours later it was midnight and I found myself with about a dozen people, mostly guys. My plan was to go to Watergate, one of the nearby techno clubs, but I didn't think that we would get in. For some reason, the others thought my presence alone would be enough to get all of us into the club — "You're a cool guy. You'll surely get us in!"

It didn't quite work out like that, though. The doorman had a look at us, singled out me and three others, saying that the four of us would get in, but the others couldn't join us. This was a rather awkward scene, but you've got to have your priorities straight, and all the hanger-ons we gained throughout the night then left us again.

In short, either go out on your own or with guys who not only understand what you're doing, but who have the same interest as you. Going out on your own isn't much of a problem either. If you go to some club often enough, you'll make friends, i.e. guys who like to say hi and who want to have some pointless conversation with you.

Girls don't mind either. Some may curiously ask where your friends are. If you're insecure, tell her that they're around here somewhere, that they left already, or that you've lost them. However, it's perfectly fine to say that you're on your own. I don't think I ever got a negative reaction to that. Quite the contrary, some girls said they wished they had the confidence to go out on their own as well, implying that they felt restrained by their friends.

A note on substances

When people think of night clubs and bars, they often assume that you have to smoke, drink, or take drugs. This is certainly not the case. I don't drink, I don't smoke, and I don't do drugs. I do not intend to patronize you, though. What you do with your life is entirely up to you, and if drugs are irresistible to you, then I assume that you are old enough to weigh their benefits and disadvantages.

People frequently ask me why I don't drink, but more out of curiosity, and not to make fun of me. You wouldn't believe how often people asked me whether others won't react weirdly if you remain sober. The reason why I don't indulge in those earthly pleasures is simply that they cloud my judgment, at the very least. In larger doses alcohol may make you quite obnoxious, too.

Keeping a clear head is not only useful because it allows you to react quickly if an opportunity presents itself to you. By the time Joe with four beers in his stomach realizes that the girl smiling ten feet away from him might be interested, some other guy could easily have beaten him to the punch already. If you don't drink, or don't do drugs, you remain in control.

Another problem is that if you drink or do drugs, you waste the entire next day to recover. On the other hand, if you take a nap before heading out, have fun for a couple of hours, and maybe pull a girl home, you'll still be functional, not only to perform in the bedroom, but also to get some things done the next day. During the week you'll probably be rested enough to power through a day at work, if your office has flextime and allows you to come in a bit later.

It's a wide spectrum between being a teetotaler and getting wasted whenever you can. If you want to wean yourself off alcohol, maybe try alternating alcoholic and non-alcoholic beverages. This is for people who feel uncomfortable not having a bottle or a glass in their hands. Alternatively, you could try to limit yourself to one drink an hour. If you stay out for two hours, this means two beers. Even on a longer night out you won't get drunk as quickly. Even better, you might slowly learn to enjoy yourself without or with much less alcohol.

People often say that they need one or two beers to warm up, and to overcome inhibitions. Interestingly, this is a psychological effect. As research has confirmed, people "compensate for the expected effects of the alcohol" by acting as if they were drunk already.[2] In other words, people become more outgoing and active *before* alcohol could have had any physiological effect on them.

You don't need alcohol to overcome your inhibitions, but it may be hard to argue about this with your regular Joe who ritually gets wasted on the weekend. Hitting on girls when sober may be quite intimidating to guys, and if you don't want to work on overcoming this mental bar-

[2]Testa M. Fillmore M. Norris J, et al. Understanding alcohol expectancy effects: revisiting the placebo condition (symposium) *Alcoholism: Clinical and Experimental Research.* 2006; 30:339–348.

rier, then a couple of beers are a suitable shortcut. Further, I don't want to ignore the fact that getting drunk and hooking up is probably the most common way of meeting girls. Surely you've heard stories from male or female friends, saying that they woke up in someone else's bed, not knowing where they were, and whether sex had actually occurred. Sometimes you may be pleasantly surprised, but you hopefully agree that this is a somewhat random approach to dating, and that there are more systematic ways to go about it.

High-level Strategies

Planning a night out

In any bigger city you'll have a good selection of clubs. But which one to go to first? If you want to maximize your return on investment, both in terms of money and time, then think of two or three clubs, and first go to the one club you like best. Some people like the idea of going from one place to another, culminating in their favorite club. Apparently they think they would miss out on something otherwise.

However, if the club you're currently at is busy already and the atmosphere good, it won't get so much better. In the best case you'll end up in a comparable place — after standing in the queue and paying cover charge again. In the worst case you'll realize that the other place was better. Therefore, stay and make the best of it if it's a good night. Leave only if you really don't get anywhere with the ladies, or if there are no attractive women around.

Knowing when to leave a venue is a good skill to develop, though. Have you ever been to a club that was dead? You arrived, and there were only a few dozen people there, even though it was midnight already. What did you do then? Some people prefer to stay and while away a couple of hours in a club in which it is almost guaranteed that nothing is going to happen. They have paid cover charge. Therefore, they want to get their money's worth, and stay.

Economists call this the *sunk cost fallacy*. The money is already spent and you're not going to get any of it back. So you might as well do something else with your time, which you find to be more enjoyable. This phenomenon is rather common. Some people force themselves to finish reading a novel they don't like, because they've invested a few dozen hours already. Others sit through a dreadfully boring movie in the cinema instead of walking out. Just don't let this happen to you. If the night genuinely sucks, then it's better to move on.

Ideally, you'll have two to three clubs in mind, and first go to the one you expect to be best. Show up before the night gets too busy, because waiting in line for two hours probably isn't your idea of fun. This is where living in a big city pays enormous dividends, since they normally all have at least one district with a high density of clubs and bars, which makes it very convenient to get from one place to the next. A strategy I used in Shoreditch and Soho in London was to go to the coolest place I knew first. If the night didn't go particularly well, I simply moved on to the next place, which was close by. In fact, going to a string of many smaller places in a row is a rather viable strategy, if they are all within walking distance. Normally it is more efficient to go to one or two bigger clubs, though.

Checking out the place

Some concepts dreamt up by the commercial pickup industry have acquired questionable fame, such as the so-called three-second rule. It says that once you see a woman, you should wait no longer than three seconds before you approach her. In practical terms it supposedly means that you shouldn't hesitate to walk up to a woman you like. However, what do you do if you are in a big club and haven't scoped out the venue yet? There is some merit to the idea of not hitting on the first semi-attractive woman you see, but on the most attractive one of a reasonably-sized subset of all the women in the club instead. If this doesn't go anywhere, you can then move further down the ladder until you've exhausted your options, meaning that there are no women left who turn you on.

Some guys literally stare at women. This is even worse when they never approach any girl at all. It's fine to have a look around first, as long as you're eventually going to interact with girls in the club. There is a nifty solution, too, if you want to follow my advice and check out what's on the menu. Instead of directly focussing on particular women, you do your own thing and don't react to your environment.

It may be difficult to describe, but I'm sure you can figure it out: Imagine you are in the corner of the dance floor in a big club. It's too crowded to get a decent overview, so you fixate on the DJ and slowly make your way through the crowd. Don't look around, or left or right, but use your peripheral vision to get an overview. Traversing the dance floor once or twice in a more or less straight line should be enough to get a good impression of where the hot girls are.

If you think this is creepy, then try it and you'll realize that it's no problem at all. Of course, in a smaller club you don't have to bother with any of this. Just get a drink at the bar, and have a look around from there. Normally the bar is conveniently located, and gives you a good overview of the venue.

In any case, don't focus too much on what other people are doing when you're in the club. There are often guys who feel uncomfortable looking around the place all the time, until they find something to focus on. This makes them look nervous, and they certainly don't look confident either. Really, it is perfectly fine to do nothing at all. Go to the bar, get a drink, and lean against the counter. If you don't know where to look, look towards the DJ booth and bop your head to the music. The guys right next to you are doing the same anyway.

Logistics

Okay, you're now at the club, you like the vibe, and there seem to be plenty of hot girls around. Now, before you get too eager and chase after the first nice pair of tits you see, relax a little bit. Take your time and explore the club first, if you're not familiar with its layout. This will save a lot of time later on.

Knowing about the layout of the venue will make your hook-ups more efficient. You furthermore might be able to capitalize on opportunities you'd otherwise needlessly waste. If you know where the dark corners are, you can easily finger a girl to an orgasm there. She may even spontaneously go down on you. None of this would happen if you didn't know the venue well.

It's one thing to take a girl directly to a spot where you can, well, get to know her a bit better, versus dragging her around the club, looking for a quiet area, or any spot to make out with her without being disturbed by her friends. It also helps you because it plays into a typical female fantasy. You sweep her off her feet, and she'll later on say that "things just happened so fast".

You should know where the doors are and where they lead to. Finding an unlocked door to a storage room is like winning the jackpot. Also, you should be aware of where the bouncers are, and where you'll find the restrooms. This isn't just important if you want to attempt to bang her in a bathroom stall, but also for practical purposes, like when you need to urinate and end up in the queue to the main restrooms because you're not aware that in some other area you'd find a bathroom that is much less busy. If this seems self-evident to you, then tell this to all the people who engage in that kind of behavior.

Related to bathrooms are bathroom attendants. Some clubs don't have them, and the best clubs have unisex bathrooms. The worst have attendants who expect a bribe to let you use a bathroom with a female friend of yours, or they'll simply keep you from doing anything naughty. This is something you'll only learn the hard way, i.e. when some dude physically keeps you from entering a bathroom stall with some girl in tow.

Staircases are also good to know. They are often places to mingle, and you may be able to just sit down with her and talk. Depending on the club and the kind of staircase, it can be much nicer than shouting into her ear on the dance floor or at the bar. Lastly, you should also know where the bars and dance floors are, but that's obvious.

Don't forget the outside area either. There may be a dark alley around the corner, or a playground, or even a dumpster behind which you'll find some privacy. You can have fun on parking lots as well. None of this is particularly romantic, but if your choice is between not getting laid and laying her down on the hood of a car and getting it over and done with in a couple of minutes, then the latter is probably preferable for both you and her. On the weekend some guy bends her over behind a dumpster, but that colleague from work has to take her to three expensive dinner dates before she might give him a hand job. In what kind of world are we living?

You can use everything but you have to know it's there! Even if you think that this is overkill, you might regret your negligence if you end up with a girl who is really into you but who has got friends with her who just won't allow her to leave with you. Yet, they normally don't mind her going for a smoke for fifteen minutes or so. Such a time window, in combination with a good knowledge of the layout of the venue and its surroundings, might be all you need.

Women throughout the night

Working a club would be smoother if everybody showed up at the exact same time. All the people would be in the mood to party at the same time, and they would be having fun at the same time, too, making it easier to interact with people. This is not how things are in reality, though. If a club opens at 10 p.m., which is quite common in London, and you show up at midnight, then some people are heading home already, while others are just arriving, but there is hopefully also a small group that is the life of the party.

If you're used to Berlin nightlife, then going out at 10 p.m. sounds ludicrous to you, given that many clubs open at midnight, and that it's common to not go to a club before 2 a.m. In London, on the other hand, most clubs will be open at 10 p.m. Some even start at 8 p.m., only opening the bar first. I really like that, because it means that if you show up at 10.30 p.m. the venue is already packed and pumping, due to so many people who come early, possibly after drinking in a pub down the road, and now wanting to have a great time in the club.

A big part of that crowd are young professionals, fresh out of university, but you also bump into girls in their last or second-to-last year of high school who have to go home before midnight or 1 a.m. Those clubs provide a rather accelerated environment. People get sucked into the atmosphere, and the main crowd, mostly students, that arrives at around midnight is ready to join a party that is already going great. With a girl from that crowd you could therefore leave rather quickly.

Let's me now generalize the previous description, and also simplify my assumptions. Say there are three waves of people. You've got the early crowd, then those who show up when most others show up, and the latecomers. The early crowd might even queue up before the place actually opens. In really popular clubs, showing up early is often the only way to get in, but this might still entail wasting a lot of time in the queue. I don't think that queuing is inherently fun, which is why I recommend going to a club once the initial crowd is inside.

It often works well to show up some time after the club has opened its doors. Just make sure you arrive before the next big heap of people arrives. Ideally, this means that you won't have to spend any time in the queue. As an added bonus there will then be plenty of people inside, including some girls who are already eager to hook up with someone. There are places where there is always a queue, often an artificial one because the club owners want to give the impression that their place is more popular than it really is.

While I recommend showing up an hour or two after the club has opened its doors, some people prefer a different strategy and instead appear in the last hour. This can work very well, too, but it has some downsides. First, in some clubs you'll still pay full cover charge, even though they are closing in an hour, which you might consider a rip-off. Further, plenty of people will have left already, so you could well have to deal with a drunk and more aggressive crowd. You might get lucky and find the occasional girl who is eager to hook up and a bit more outgoing because most of her friends have left already. Well, just give it a try. I don't think that clubs are that much fun at the end of the night, but with a bit of luck you can get laid rather easily.

What I wrote above was just to give you a general idea about how a typical night out is structured. Of course there is some overlap between the groups. Some people come early and stay all night long, so it was by no means an exhaustive enumeration. What I would recommend in general, once you've gotten a good feel for the mood people are in, is to proceed more systematically. Consider hitting on girls when you feel that the night has really started, and a good part of the crowd seem to be enjoying themselves. If you are more perceptive, figure out where the person or group in question is at and act accordingly.

For instance, don't try to pull a girl that just arrived and is still freezing because it was cold outside. Also, I would not focus too much on women who still look a bit uptight. They are clutching to the strap of their handbag, or holding on to the hand of their girlfriend, and looking around in an insecure manner. At this point they normally aren't ready to get picked up yet.

To tell you another one of my war stories, I once had a girl say to me that she thought I was hot, but that it was way too early to leave with me, because she had just arrived. To them it obviously doesn't matter that you've been in the venue for two hours already. Sure, if you were exactly the kind of guy she is looking for, or she desperately wants to get laid, then it's possible to pull a girl basically the moment she walks in, but those are rare exceptions. I once left with a girl I chatted up while she was queuing at the coat check, and walked straight out with her a few minutes after she had entered the club. Things like this might happen to you, but you shouldn't expect them to happen.

Girls have to loosen up, too. Consequently, if she just walked into the place she probably won't be up for some finger banging in a dark corner five minutes later. This is not necessarily because she needs to be hammered to engage in that kind of activity, even though this is a common misconception people have when they think about clubs. Instead, people have to get into the right mood before they are able to enjoy themselves in the club. Clubs are not part of real life. They provide a form of escapism, which takes some time to get used to. This applies to all but the most veteran partygoers, who have a hard time adjusting to regular life instead.

Another problem is that normally you're not the guy of her dreams, but pretty acceptable. She might go for you if nothing better comes along. I know that this doesn't sound flattering, but that's the reality of picking up girls. In that regard, I'd like to share another story. I was talking to some girl at one of the bars at Berghain, and things were going great. It was rather early in the night — not even 1 a.m., which is to say that it was quite early for a techno club in Berlin.

I thought that she was ready to leave with me, but she suddenly became a bit skeptical when I suggested we leave the place, so she consulted her girlfriend. The verdict I received was damning. Her friend said, "I think he's cute, but isn't it really early?", implying that she might get someone hotter if she just waited a bit longer. I don't know how her night ended, but I saw her two hours later sitting at the bar all by herself when I was on the way to the exit with some other girl. That's also a lesson for guys: don't always expect that there will be someone better. If you find her attractive, then make the interaction count, or otherwise don't bother with her at all.

Meeting Women

Do you just want to get laid?

With experience, guys tend to grow out of the need to count the number of girls they have had sex with. Yet, I do understand that a big draw of going to clubs is the prospect of sex. If you are more of a beginner in the field of seduction, your motivation may well be to have sex with a lot of girls. Feel free to pursue this goal, but heed my warning that it won't be quite like you imagine. The first few one-nights stands are probably exciting. Once it becomes repetitive, though, you will be much better off looking for women who could play a bigger role in your life. A one-night stand may be a bad investment of your time, but if it leads to a fling, it's a pretty decent pay-off. But let's assume you aren't there yet and just want to get laid.

Sitting in your easy chair and wondering how to get laid with the least effort, you may come up with the idea of going for average-looking girls. You know the kind of girl I'm talking about: not particularly good-looking, but good enough so that you would likely get hard. You probably wouldn't make out with her in public, but you wouldn't feel completely embarrassed if your friends saw you with her. In other words, some plain Jane.

This idea may theoretically make sense. Unfortunately, too many men think like that and therefore that kind of woman finds herself with no shortage of suitors. It's quite obvious if you think about it some more. Less attractive girls don't get approached much because they aren't sexually attractive enough, and many men don't dare to approach the better looking girls because they think that she probably has boyfriend anyway or that she is out of their league.

What I find so fascinating is that sometimes the most average-looking women have the nastiest of personalities and think they are so very good-looking, largely because they don't grasp that they are seen as an easier target by guys. They may even have a greater number of guys coming after them than much more attractive women whom many guys are intimidated by. You'll often find that good-looking girls are much friendlier, even when they are not interested, than the domesticated pig in high heels standing next to her.

In the end, the paradoxical situation is that it can be quite difficult to pull average-looking girls because they have too many guys chasing after them. You may even witness situations where guys talk to the plain Janes, and ignore her hot friend who is therefore forced to fiddle with her smartphone to make herself look busy. This is also what makes good-looking women look aloof, and it's not even their fault. It's more like a curse.

Categories of women

Generally, go for women you find attractive, and who are somewhat similar to you. If you followed the advice in the preceding chapters, you have done some soul-searching to find out what you really like, and have begun styling yourself in a particular way. If you have now turned into a hipster, you'll be hanging out in hipster clubs and hipster bars, hitting on hipster chicks. Anything else would be a waste of your resources.

However, people are not quite so one-dimensional. As a guy you can still successfully pull off the aging hipster look — I think I've done that with pretty decent success. On the other hand, for women this is much more difficult to achieve, simply because they age much faster. Also, because girls are a strong currency without which clubs targeting a heterosexual crowd wouldn't function so well, the door policy is normally much more restrictive towards guys. Young women, as long as they are at least mildly attractive, normally have little difficulty getting into any place.

Consequently, while you and your hipster buddies hang out at the bar, you might notice that the crowd is somewhat diverse. This was to be expected. You graduated from a guy who was just there to one of the attractions of the venue. This doesn't mean that you can only hit on hipster girls. Let's say of the ten attractive hipster girls in the venue, you've banged two already, the third one turned you down last time, and the others all know those girls, each other, and you. Does this mean that it's slim pickings today for Joe Hipster?

No, not at all. Instead, you make a selection from the rest of the crowd. Therefore, let's go through what else you might find among the non-hipster crowd in your favorite club. Note that the following classification is to be understood as a rough outline. The categories I'm about to introduce often overlap. The guiding principle is still that you should generally only go after girls you find attractive, and not bother with their unattractive friends. Go for what you want, and not for girls you find less attractive just because you believe they are easier to get. For instance, when you see a woman who is out on her own, I presume that if you're going to talk to her, it's because you find her attractive, and not because you assume, quite rightly so, that she's looking for dick. In a way, all women in the club are.

I'll continue with this example: yes, women who go out on their own, sometimes referred to as lone wolves, are normally eager to get laid. They seem to specifically look for a one-night stand, possibly even a quickie in the bathroom stall. Those women normally are a bit older, at least in their late 20s. They might have a loving boyfriend or husband who is temporarily out of town, or maybe she's in town for a conference and snuck away from her colleagues for an hour or two — so that she can cheat on her husband or boyfriend.

Being potentially more mature, those women tend to know what they want, and they won't waste your time, no matter whether they are interested in you or not. If she's not, she'll let you know about it quickly. On the other hand, if she is, she might discreetly rub your crotch and ask whether you'd like to go for a walk. Since those women respect your time, you should do likewise and not waste theirs either.

Related to lone wolves are the clichéd cougars, i.e. more mature women, either on their own or in groups. Those do indeed exist outside of TV shows and movies. In groups I find them hard to tolerate, as I've found that they are generally on the same level as groups of teenage girls, if not worse. That might just be a general feature of all-female groups in the night life, no matter their age, though. In this group you'll meet your fair share of recent divorcées and single mothers. I would recommend to not bother with those women at all, but if you must, I'll let you know that, yes, they should be much easier to get, since they've grown out of playing games.

Cougars can't much afford to play games anymore because they realize that they can't compete so well against women who are one or two decades younger than them. They are fully aware of this, which is also why they often opt to get cosmetic surgery done. Breast implants are a quick fix to get attention from guys again, and while they are at it, they'll have some work on their lips done, their nose straightened, and their tummy tucked, too. Despite certain corners in the mainstream media proclaiming how confident and desirable older women are, the women affected know all too well that they used to be much more appealing to members of the opposite sex.

Depending on your age, lone wolves and cougars might not be your first choice, though. If you're in your early to mid-twenties, you'll probably be looking for girls who are at most your age. Those girls are still young. They have nice bodies to show off, if they take care of themselves. Indeed, if you notice a woman who shows a lot of skin, you can safely assume that she's looking to score. In the same vein, hair extensions, excessive make-up, or attention-seeking clothing are all giveaways. No, this doesn't mean that she'll hop on any cock that comes her way, but you can reasonably assume that she's a bit more eager than she would be on other days of the month.

This is an aspect where the possibly lower level of maturity of younger girls comes into play, because often those girls tend to drink a bit more as well. This means that, on the one hand, you're dealing with a girl who is eager to hook up, but on the other she might be quite a pain in the neck to deal with, due to alcohol or substance abuse. Even if they aren't necessarily drunk, they may nonetheless act in a rather uncontrollable way. I once had a girl who was dancing in hot pants and a top that showed some underboob climb on my shoulders and flail her arms around as she was shouting the lyrics of the song that was playing. Sure, you can pull those girls home, but they are a bit of a headache. If you find them difficult to deal with, then it might be better for your mental health to go for other girls instead.

Lastly, it is often rather easy to go after women who look as if they don't go out a lot. After a break-up, the first thing an insecure girl who wants to rebuild her self-esteem does is go through three or four guys before she starts dating again. Don't ask me about the underlying logic. It's just an observation. However, after having been in a relationship with Joe Average for a few months or a couple of years, she has stopped going out for a while and lost touch with fashion trends. If she hasn't developed a clear identity before, she will therefore look a bit out of place in the club. Should you happen to notice this, you've got a head start over your competition. But keep in mind that her flirting skills might be a bit rusty, which means that unlike the other girls she probably needs a bit more time.

Without wanting to go into this in too much detail, I would recommend that with women who look as if they don't go out much, you should try to find out a few things about her first. I've met some real head cases from that category. To give you a few examples: after talking to some girl for a few minutes and feeling her up, she said that if she goes home with me, she expects me to become her boyfriend. Another asked me, while we were waiting for our serving of street food, how many children I wanted to have. Some other woman seemed more sane at first, until I had her lying in front of me, legs spread, only to lunge forward, rip the condom off my cock and telling me that she wants to do it without. This was enough to make me steer clear of that category of women, instead preferring the usual young hipster girls.

A smarter way to approach

When guys were going out with me, they noticed that I was approaching only very few girls, and that those interactions tended to go very well. It virtually never happened that a girl shot me down. This led to two kinds of questions. The less experienced guys asked me whether I could get any girl I wanted, because they see me hitting on two or three a night, making out with the first, the second at least being friendly, and the third leaving with me. However, the more experienced guys asked how I knew that she was interested in me.

If you spend some time going out, you will notice that many guys, particularly when they are in groups of two, approach girls more or less randomly. Sometimes, this leads to a rather negative reception, other girls ignore them, and sometimes they meet girls who at first tolerate them. Then they stick to them for the rest of the night, and the girls think the guys are kind of okay and tolerate them, too. At the end of the night it's still not a sealed deal, and the girls might just disappear, hoping that they'll meet some more appealing guys next weekend.

Thus, you could to what those allegedly normal guys are doing, which is throwing mud at the wall, hoping that some of it will stick. Alternatively, you could try my much more analytical approach, which I'm going to outline over the next few sections. Note that people have called me a sociopath when I detailed my approach, while some women have asked me whether they had "fuck me" written on their forehead, because they found it hard to grasp that I read them like an open book and had sex with them within half an hour. Apparently it's not considered normal in our society to reflect over what you are doing. Read on if engaging in supposedly sociopathic behavior sounds tempting to you. Otherwise, feel free to keep fumbling your way to sex.

Female signals

Only in rare cases do women signal clearly that they are interested in a particular man. Normally, you can at best hope for mixed signals. This is largely due to culture. In Western society it's the man's task to approach the woman, while the woman doesn't want to be seen as easy. On the other hand, she also doesn't want to feel the negative emotions that may come with rejection. So, instead of smiling for half a minute at a guy she fancies, she will only glance over, and maybe flick her hair, hoping that he will respond to this. Some women won't even do that and instead expect you to read their mind, which is why I recommend the mentality I describe in a later section, Testing the waters.

The reason for mixed signals is that they allow the girl to say to herself that she wasn't really interested if you end up ignoring her, which helps her to maintain her self-esteem. On the other hand, if you walk up to her and ask her how she's doing, it's obvious to anybody that you're not just being social. If she reacts coldly, you can of course claim that you were not really interested in her, but apparently you were interested enough in her to try your luck. This isn't quite so comfortable as the situation the girl is in.

In the opposite scenario, where the girl likes you, and eventually hooks up with you, her strategy further helps her to maintain a positive self-image. It's one thing for a girl to give every schmuck in the bar fuck me eyes, and quite another if she gives off subtle signals here and there, and then takes some guy home. It then all just happened. You know, she only went to the bar to hang out with her friends, and not to meet some guy to have a one-night stand with. Even if she repeats this week after week, she'll keep viewing herself as daddy's good girl.

Women don't want to be held accountable for their actions, which is reflected in their dating strategies. Even among more promiscuous women it's quite rare that any would say that she loves to fuck random dudes. Instead, they say they've had a lot of boyfriends or, slightly more ambiguous, that they have many male friends. In fact, those are the same lies girls tend to tell themselves when they're seeing a guy who is only interested in sex.

Why women go out

Another lie women tell themselves and others is that they don't go out to get laid or to find their knight in shining armor. "No, we're just socializing!", they protest. But let's be real here! While it is apparently completely okay to accuse guys of only going out to get laid, it's sacrilege if you point out that women do the same. Let's therefore have a look at how plausible their claim is.

Just remember the last time you saw two girls, or a handful of girls, in a club, pretending to socialize. If clubs and bars in your city are anything like the ones I know, then your typical girl did the following before she appeared on the dance floor, gyrating her ass in front of you:

- she took a shower

- she meticulously fixed her hair

- she spent about an hour picking the right clothes to wear

- … and matching shoes

- … and complementary jewelry

- … and applied make-up to complete her look

- … and pondered over the right perfume

- … and took a dozen selfies

- she went from her place to the club, involving walking, cab fare, or some time on public transport

- she did wait in line, but she's happy when the doorman allows her to skip it

- she might have paid cover charge

- she now pays inflated prices for beverages

- she messes up her biorhythm by staying up much longer than usual

This wasn't a particularly creative list, and you surely could fit in other items, like spending time online to listen to the music of this or that hot new DJ to help her decide where to go to, or incessantly chatting with her girlfriends before heading out. The point, though, is that all of this is an awful lot of effort if the purpose was just to socialize with their friends.

Most girls go out in packs, so wherever they came from they could just have stayed and socialized there. However, they much rather go where guys can hit on them. True, she might not want to jump on any Tom, Dick, and Harry's cock, but she surely loves the attention she's getting. One of the favorite activities of better-looking girls who lack self-esteem is to complain to her girlfriends about all the guys who are hitting on her, particularly if her girlfriend doesn't get a lot of attention from guys.

Girls go out to meet guys. Sure, dancing awkwardly in high heels, socializing, and getting wasted are also part of the equation, but I'm fairly certain that if the prospect of meeting some cool guy wasn't important to them we would have women-only clubs, catering to heterosexual women, so that they could do all the socializing they wanted with each other, without being disturbed by men, just like we have women-only gyms and fitness classes.

If women only wanted to hang out with their friends, they could be much more efficient about it. When I want to talk to one of my friends, I call him, and if we want to hang out, then this can be arranged rather easily, without involving any of the steps I've just mentioned, and any of the mental acrobatics that only serve to provide a pretense.

It's apparently too much for a lot of girls to admit that they indeed like it when guys hit on them. In the best case they get laid by some hunk, and in the worst case they still get the gratification of shooting down some loser. There aren't many places where an attractive girl can trade a bit of time for copious amounts of attention, and if she ends up having sex with someone, it can be chalked up as something that just happened.

Specific versus general interest

If you are interested in a particular woman, you can always just walk up to her and see how it goes. If it doesn't go anywhere, you simply move on. It might happen that she pretends to be cold and strong and oh-so-in-control, but warms up once you say hi. There are also cases where she acts in a disinterested manner, yet willingly goes along with everything, and turns into the sweetest thing after you've made her come. I'm tempted to say that such women have serious issues, but it's good to have the experience.

More commonly, though, girls will give some kind of indication of how interested they are. It may be very subtle, such that she walks a bit slower as she passes you. One of the more humorous variations of that theme I witnessed was when a girl stopped, turned a little bit, and pretended to wipe something off her shoes. Meanwhile, she fully stretched her legs, so that I could check out her ass. Others rub their tits against your chest as they're walking past, or their ass against your crotch. I wouldn't call those moves subtle anymore, but some guys even miss that. Those signals are directed at you in particular. Maybe there are cases where this is indeed accidental, but I don't think I ever encountered one.

One signal that means that she is particularly interested in you is eye contact. Some women make eye contact with one or two guys, hoping that one of them will make a move. Others look around and flick her hair a few times. Both are perfectly valid strategies. The problem, though, is that plenty of men find direct signals intimidating, and when they notice general signals, they think they don't mean anything.

Likewise, a girl dancing seductively might just want the attention of the crowd. However, if she walks over to where you and your buddy stand, and turns so that her ass is directly facing your loins, then it's normally an invitation for you to check her out and make a move, provided you like what you see.

A girl showing general interest is not interested in talking to anybody specific. Instead, she wants to entice guys to hit on her. Such girls look around the venue, don't always huddle with their best friend but instead stand slightly further away so that you can check her out, or close her eyes and flick her hair a few times, hoping that she'll get noticed. Your chances aren't quite as good in those instances. However, you certainly shouldn't wait too long either. More often than not she may go home with the first best guy who comes along. It might be you, but if you first head to the bar to get some liquid courage, it may very well be someone else instead.

Subtle signals

Women normally aren't especially forward. Sure, in a busy night club it may happen that a woman pinches your ass or squeezes your junk as she walks past. As a man you normally wouldn't do that without having been given a clear indication that such strong moves were desired. Instead of women hitting on you, they wait for you to make a move. As you might know, women tend to be insecure and want to avoid the risk of rejection. Therefore, they place the burden of the approach firmly on your shoulders. You don't have to be too intimidated, though. It might take some courage to approach women, but recognizing the right signals goes a long way.

Not all women are comfortable displaying sexual interest clearly. Normally it's a minority of women who dare to flick their long hair or dance seductively to music. It's also the case that those women often merely want attention. Those who want to hook up tend to be a bit more discreet. For instance, they may look over briefly. Just looking over itself doesn't mean much. Some dating guides fantasize about a scenario in which the woman first looks at you, and when you notice her, she'll quickly look away. If she then seeks eye contact again, this is to be understood as a clear signal.

Reality isn't necessarily that formal, though. What often happens is that a woman looks at you because she is curious. It doesn't mean that she is willing to jump on your dick right away. Yet, if you like her, then walk up to her. Some women then get quite nervous and look down, while facing your direction. I perceive this as a submissive gesture. Then walk up to her and say hi. On the other hand, if she turns her head in a different direction or, worse, turns around so that her back faces you, then you've probably read too much into her brief glance. Feel free to persist, but don't be surprised if you won't get anywhere.

Especially in clubs that aren't busy yet, you can notice

that some women will move a bit closer when walking past. This does not mean that she will brush her tits against you, though. What sometimes also happens is that they not only move a bit closer as they walk past, but walk a little bit slower, so that you can check them out a bit longer. It doesn't necessarily stop there, as sometimes she may then correct her posture and stick her chest out. If all of this doesn't get your attention, she may then stop, pull out her phone, and pretend to read a text message, all while standing straight, taking some deep breaths, and flexing her ass cheeks. All of this is not so subtle if you pay attention to your surroundings.

Yes, women who are more sexually aggressive will brush their tits against you. Those you can simply stop, and depending on her mood, you may end up making out with her right away. More reserved women won't do that, though. In their mind, the mere fact that they are walking past *you*, and not someone else, is an invitation for you to approach them.

Sexual motivation

Guys with little to no sexual experience sometimes have the bizarre idea that any woman would be good enough for them. You can hear similar sentiments from guys who are going through a long dry spell. There might be guys who are willing to fuck literally anything, but I don't think that this will do them any favors. True, by acting like that you might get more notches on your bedpost, but would you think back on all those women with a sense of pride or achievement? More likely than not, you'd rather forget about them.

Sexual confidence hardly comes from having sex with women you're not attracted to. What good is it if you have to swallow a couple of blue pills just so that you can get hard? Your body might be telling you something when your penis refuses to serve you. True, not all women look like supermodels, centerfolds, or porn stars, but there are plenty of attractive women around.

You probably won't find the perfect woman for you, but you will encounter enough women you find attractive. Let's say you really like legs. Obesity rates are skyrocketing, but since all it takes for a girl to have attractive legs is a bit of exercise and a modicum of restraint when she's passing the cookie jar, you'll find plenty to like. I've been told that some guys like girls with big asses. Well, there certainly are plenty of those around, so go ahead and enjoy yourself! Similarly, if you have strong physical response towards brunettes — as long as the hair color is right and they are at least mildly attractive — you'll find plenty, too.

Finding some girl for any kind of short-term relationship is not such a big challenge. Only once you're looking towards settling down with someone will you realize how very few women are out there who would make for a good partner. But if you're not interested in that then just go for what you want and make sure you use protection.

Should you pursue this strategy you'll realize that interacting with women is a lot more fun because you're genuinely interested in them. This interest may initially only be sexual, like hers, but at least there is undeniable sexual interest. Women notice that, too, just as you notice when a girl seems to be sexually interested in you. This is a much healthier situation than trying to get laid at all costs.

I tend to think it's also a more successful strategy, even though this might sound paradoxical to some. The reason is simply that you'll be more motivated if you're at least a bit horny for her, and if she likewise wants you, then things can happen rather quickly. The result is a more fulfilling sex life. Further, you'll also get to build sexual confidence because if you go for what you want and happen to get a few of those girls, you'll get all the satisfaction that comes from having sex with girls you desire, and who also crave your cock.

Sexual excitement

Building upon the last section I would like to drive home the point that sexual excitement, horniness, is a great motivating force for picking up girls. If you're talking to a girl you hardly feel attracted to you might find yourself debating in your head whether you really should take her home. I certainly remember situations where I walked down to my favorite bar and happened to bump into a girl who seemed keen on getting with me, while

I was relatively lukewarm towards her. In such a situation you'll ask yourself whether you should appreciate the fact that she makes it easy for you, and go for somewhat mechanical sex. The alternative is of course to ignore her advances.

I can understand guys who jump at those opportunities. At the very least you know that she's into you, which will make sex a lot more enjoyable than between two people who would both rather fuck someone else. Just think about it: you end up talking to that girl that looks okay, and she is getting really touchy-feely. You'll probably get a bit horny too, won't you? After all, if you felt absolutely no sexual attraction, you would probably have walked off when she rubbed your thighs and accidentally let her fingers run over your crotch.

If a girl you initially thought was only mildly attractive seems to be really into you, you might find yourself being attracted to her as well, at least a little bit. There surely are limitations, but if she's okay-looking, you'll probably experience this. Even more interesting is that this works both ways. She might at first think that you're just some okay-looking guy, but if she's sexually available and you happen to fit her bill at least somewhat, you might find that she'll respond positively to you.

Of course she could wait and hope that some guy who looks like a Greek god will pull her, but most likely her expectation will be that, of the many guys who will hit on her that night, she won't like quite a few because they aren't her type. Then there are guys who are too obnoxious or, with some girls, not obnoxious enough. But it's getting late and so far Prince Charming has stood her up yet again. On the other hand, there is you. Well, you're not super-hot, but you look quite okay, and you seem to really want her. This could be motivation enough for her to go home with you.

Depending on your level of experience and your perception, those descriptions may sound rather foreign to you, but just keep paying attention. Maybe make it a rule to only approach women you feel genuinely attracted to, and see what happens. You will probably notice that even though you're approaching a much smaller number of women, your success rate is a lot higher, and the quality of the interactions a lot better.

Capitalizing on opportunities

You would have to be an astonishingly good-looking guy for women to do all the work. If this does not apply to you (it certainly doesn't apply to me), then you will have to lead the interaction all the way to sex, wherever it may take place. How successful you'll be with women depends not just on how you look and how many available women there are around you. A lot boils down to how persistent you are, and whether you are willing to close the deal.

You may have heard of statistics according to which the average Joe has sex with seven women in his lifetime.

Needless to say, that's not a lot. If you want to push the envelope, you can reach that number in two months with a bit of luck. If you want to go overboard and happen to be in the right environment, it's a matter of about two weeks.

There is a difference between having opportunities and making the most of them. Only rarely have I met guys who've had many opportunities and made the best of them. Plenty of guys get countless opportunities and basically let them all slide. It seems that the better looking guys sometimes make less of an effort. Granted, they don't need to work as hard. However, when I was talking to some of those guys, I was often surprised at how little experience with women they had. All they needed was just to be a little bit more aggressive. If you are in this position, then your problems might all be solved within a few weekends.

But what if you don't look that good? Well, if you've maximized your looks and you're putting yourself in a position where you can meet women relatively easily, you should experience at least some success. You should not be complacent and expect the women to come to you. Instead, you have to make an active effort, and if needed, approach a few more women than you otherwise would, or stay out an hour longer than you had originally planned. Of course, once a woman is interested, you have to be willing to go all the way and do your best to take her home — instead of hemming and hawing and hoping that you'll end up in her bedroom somehow.

Make it a habit to talk to women you find attractive! This takes just a moment, and the payoff can be tremendous. There are plenty of guys who look pretty average but simply work harder. They won't turn heads. However, because they don't let opportunities pass them by, they do much better than you'd expect. Sure, they get turned down, some rather frequently, but if they happen to come across a girl who wants to get laid and he's kind of her type, and demonstrates that he won't beat around the bush, then he'll get laid almost certainly.

No matter how you see yourself, whether you're good-looking or more average-looking: by being willing to capitalize on your opportunities you will get laid more often, in absolute terms. Being more active on a night out is certainly preferable to waiting for some lucky encounter to happen. In fact, an average-looking guy who is determined to make the most of the opportunities he's getting will have more success with women than any good-looking but indecisive guy.

Successful Approaches

Clubs are different

If you are used to meeting girls though your social circle or common activities, you'll be surprised how different it is to meet girls in clubs. Sure, you can attempt to talk to a girl in a club for hours, exchange phone numbers and hope to go on a date some days later. This is not very productive, though. What you instead should do, if you see a girl you like, is walk up to her.

You can skip any kind of introduction, no matter where you are. Let's say she's standing at the bar, waiting for her drink. You then slide up to her and, for instance, ask her how she's doing. On the dance floor you can high-five her and pull her in. Otherwise a question as stupid as, "Having fun?", said with a genuine smile, never disappoints.

Even better, because those are such simple lines, you will only get her attention if she finds you somewhat attractive. Guys who see themselves as great entertainers easily end up talking to some woman for one or two hours, not realizing that she may like listening to him, but could think of a million other things she'd rather do than fucking him.

Frankly, your conversational ability is quite irrelevant. Outside the club environment this is clearly not the case, but when people are going out, they want to have a good time first and foremost. Most don't have a good time, so they normally welcome any kind of distraction. The point of those random phrases is therefore not to launch into a deep conversation, but to evoke some kind of reaction.

Imagine a girl walked up to you, playfully knocked on your chest twice, and with a big grin on her face shouted, "Enjoying yourself?" What would you think? Your reaction would presumably almost completely depend on how attractive you find her. If she's plain average, you might just ignore her, but what if she was your type of girl? In that case, you'd reply something equally nonsensical, maybe, "Yeah, awesome night!", and take her hand, and maybe dance with her for a bit, before you dragged her off into a dark or quiet corner to make out with her.

So far, I have not spilt much ink on the specifics of approaches. I'll cover some in subsequent sections, but there really isn't so much to it. I hope you've internalized the content of the previous chapters and made some changes to your life. Do your homework, and become the kind of guy who dares to polarize. If you have some attractive qualities, i.e. qualities that are attractive to some women, you should be fine, since you no longer disappear in the crowd. Without interest from her nothing will work. It's not your words that will get you the girl, and most certainly not in clubs.

Group sizes

The by far best situation concerning group sizes is, unfortunately, one which only rarely happens, namely a woman who is out all by herself. Even prostitutes often have a colleague with them when they're scouring upscale venues for potential clients. Thus, whenever you see a woman all by herself sitting at the bar, you should strongly consider making a move.

It can be absurdly easy to pull a woman who is out on her own. The reasons for her behavior can be manifold. Yes, she only wants to hook up. But she may simply be new in the city, or was ordered by her company to go to a conference and wanted to get away from her colleagues. If you think you'll one day find the woman of your dreams sitting on a bar stool in a tight dress, suggestively sucking on a straw, you'll probably be waiting until the cows come home. On the other hand, if you're into more mature women, then stopping by at a hotel bar may well be worth it.

A fairly frequent occurrence is two girls going out, in order to have fun. Having fun normally means looking for dick. Meeting two confident girls is fantastic, because the girl who chooses you will tell the other one that everything is fine. However, groups of two can be a bit difficult to handle if one of the girls feels insecure, simply because she doesn't like the thought of being out on her own. Consequently, she may want to interfere if you're about to hit it off with her friend.

I don't want to generalize too much, but there seems to be a fundamental difference between male and female friendships. When I hang out with some guy, it's usually someone I consider to be my equal, and it's someone who is as independent as I am. On the other hand, you rarely see two really hot women going out on their own. Normally, one of the girls is a bit less attractive, to put it in polite terms. The hot girl could go out on her own, but lacks the confidence. She then has to find some other girl to go out with. However, if all her girlfriends are in a relationship, they may not want to go to a club, looking for a new guy. Thus, she'll eventually end up calling the one fat girl she barely speaks to but who is always available.

I found it quite surprising how little those women cared about their alleged friend, though. If you're quick, you can leave with the girl before her friend even notices that she's gone. Sometimes you may not even know that the girl you're with wasn't actually out on her own. I was often amused when, sitting in a cab or a night bus, the girl's phone rang and her friend wanted to know where she was. That being said, it's quite difficult to recover from a situation in the club where the unattractive friend gives your girl a speech about how egotistical she is, or how slutty it would be if she went home with you.

It's best to try to prevent that kind of interference. Just talk to the other girl if she's around, and be nice to her. Showing a little bit of respect can go a long way. She only has to tolerate you, and if she has a modicum of decency, then she'll let you hook up with her hot friend. The better behaved ones will in fact leave you alone after a while, pretending that they are getting tired or have to look after their cat.

Mixed groups of three people are quite rare but can be exceedingly easy to deal with. If you see two guys with a girl, I wouldn't expect too much. However, if you see one guy and two girls, then one of the girls is most definitely single. She is likely to be in a similar position as the girl in the previous scenario. Her best friend presumably felt pity for her, but since she's in a relationship, she didn't want to go out without her boyfriend. Thus, they all go out together, trying to make her forget that her boyfriend broke up with her weeks ago or whatnot.

Normally, you can't quite expect people to openly en-courage you to pick up some girl. Yet, in such situations it almost always happened, if the girl liked me at least a little bit. I've experienced that the couple both wanted me to take care of her friend, telling me that they think she really likes me. I even remember hearing, "Have fun, the two of you!", as I was leaving with the girl within minutes. Being the rebound guy isn't necessarily bad, but normally this role is reserved for some guy in her wider social circle.

Larger groups can be viewed as a collection of small groups. If you see a group of ten or twelve people, they are not all best friends with each other. Often, they know each other from school or work, and everybody will have one or two people in the group they like a bit more than the others. Sometimes, though, there is a hierarchy.

Particularly among larger groups of girls, there is often some alpha bitch — this term is a reference to a common trope from TV shows and movies, not some kind of insult. It may take some experience to handle such situations. What seems to work reasonably well is focusing on the girl you like, and if you're hitting it off with her, hang out with the group, and be friendly to the other girls. Eventually, you'll try to disappear with your girl, which can be the tricky part.

Girls in their mid-twenties are normally a bit more independent, but if you bump into a group of teenagers on vacation, then the alpha bitch may have too much control and keep a very close eye on you. Of course, there are situations where you end up with the leader of the female group, at which point you might witness the reverse behavior, namely that one of her underlings pesters you and your girl, which can lead to humorous scenes.

I don't think there is a general solution to that kind of problem, so I'd advise you to be nice and talk normally to any girl who attempts to interfere, instead of being confrontational. Sometimes they change their behavior after just a few sentences. However, there is no guarantee that this will work. If she's hell-bent on wrecking your pickup, she will succeed. In the worst case, she will simply cause some drama that puts all her friends in a bad mood.

Female role play

Many guys give up way too soon, not realizing when they are throwing away a perfectly good chance. Some girls love playing hard to get, and tease you a little bit. Sadly, this expression of playful resistance is too much for men who think that picking up girls should be effortless. Yet, if you view it as a ritual that only serves to increase sexual tension, it can be entertaining to play along, at least for a little while.

To give you an example, if a girl says to you, "I bet you do this all the time!", or "I don't think I should get involved with a guy like you", while she keeps touching you and looking into your eyes, then she is engaging in a role play according to which you have to pretend that you are seducing her, while she pretends that she is being seduced. In reality, seduction is a mutual process. Nothing would happen if she wasn't interested as well.

What you say in those situations is almost irrelevant. Making the rookie mistake of trying to discuss the issue, and elaborating that you are not that kind of guy only ensures that you really won't be that kind of guy. If you can't think of anything good to say, then keep your mouth shut and smirk as you keep looking into her eyes. On the other hand, if you want to respond, then drop a one-liner like, "Yes, I do this every night." As long as you don't miss a beat, you'll do fine.

I wouldn't recommend sounding too arrogant, particularly if you don't have a lot of experience. Note that if you overdo it, you can easily repel her. A safer bet is either to drily say that whatever she said might indeed be the case, or ask her rhetorically whether she's sure that she's all that different from you, as you squeeze her ass. Those are just suggestions, but they should suffice to get the idea.

Some guys walk away from the girl because they mistake flirting as resistance. However, it's even worse when guys keep engaging women who have no *sexual* interest. Surely you have found yourself talking to some girl once who seemed to really enjoy your company. You were never certain whether she was really interested, but because you didn't make a move either, she firmly put you into the dreaded friend zone, and you were wondering how to get out of there.

That is a situation you should avoid altogether, though. I don't say that you shouldn't have female friends if you feel like it, but meeting women in an asexual way and then attempting to gradually turn an interaction sexual is a plan that is doomed to failure. Instead, she should know that you're talking to her because you're sexually interested. Don't ever be afraid that if you made a move, she'd walk off. If this is what you fear, then you are only prolonging the inevitable, because sexual interest doesn't develop over time. You know that you want her when you look at her, and it's the same for her.

Testing the waters

Given that women tend to send ambiguous signals, you can't be too forward. Sure, if she stares at you, while slowly licking her lips, you can attempt a more physical approach, like putting your arm around her waist as you say hi to her. But what if you only witness some hair flicking or, worse, a girl who seems to not give much of an indication at all whether she wants to be approached? Luckily for you, she's in a club, so it's much more likely that she does indeed want to meet somebody than not.

In those instances I recommend a low-key approach. Slowly walk up to her, and pay attention to whether there is any reaction. As I wrote in the previous chapter, looking downwards, but still facing you with her body can safely be interpreted as a sign of submission. Should she abruptly look away, and turn her body, you're probably better off ditching your plan altogether.

This leaves a third possible outcome, namely that she remains neutral. In that case, keep going! It hardly matters what you said to her, because the important aspect is how she reacts to your presence. A question like "Having a fun night?" might be met with a disrespectful stare. In fact, if she shows any sign of disrespect, I would not bother at all with her. If there is greater interest, she will normally say something in return. If this is too much for you, then stand next to her and accidentally touch her, and see how she reacts. You could, for instance, move closer so that your arm touches hers. Women often accidentally press their tits against you when they are interested, so this is only par for the course.

For the more daring among you there are other options. What I consider to be eminently effective is taking her hand gently, as you say something to her — provided you have an indication that she at the very least isn't hostile towards you. Again there are three possible outcomes. She could take her hand away, which means that she needs more time or isn't interested. Sometimes you take her hand, and she squeezes it in return. This is a very good signal that should encourage you to keep going. Lastly, she could let you keep holding her hand, without showing much of a reaction. This might surprise some of you, but this is also positive feedback, because it means that she has accepted your move, and established a baseline for the interaction.

If holding her hand is too much for you, then put your arm around her. Again, there are three kinds of reaction. First, she might lean in, encouraging your to keep going, or even start touching you. Second, she might move away from you. Lastly, she could remain neutral and tolerate your touching her. Two out of these three outcomes are good.

What I'm describing here is a fairly low-risk approach, which is particularly appropriate in smaller venues. You don't want to be perceived as the guy who hits on one girl after another. With some experience you'll find ways to be very smooth about those approaches. For instance, as you order a drink at the bar, you could put your arm around the waist of the girl standing next to you and who seems interested. Do this casually, and if she doesn't like it, she'll move away.

On a related note, if you know a bit of computer science, you might be familiar with operations that are essentially without cost, sometimes referred to as *for free primitives*, because they piggyback on operations your program has to perform anyway. You can apply this theoretical concept directly to your approaches. If you want to order a drink at the bar, then doing an approach as the one I just described also essentially comes for free and, even if it doesn't go well, won't negatively affect the rest of your night.

The whole point is to give the girl a chance to react to you. Don't pay too much attention to her words, but instead focus on her physical reaction. If she accuses you of being some kind of sleazy guy, but smiles at you and undresses you with her eyes, then the last thing on your mind should be to bail on her. Conversely, if she is behaving too neutrally in the course of the interaction, you might want to consider moving on as well. While you can pull girls like that, to me it feels as if you have to drag them to the finishing line.

Conversations

Some of you are probably itching to know what you should talk about, and how you should structure a conversation with a woman. In short, it doesn't really matter. However, I would strongly advise you to not engage in any kind of controversial topic. If you go out in a particular district in your city, and have a couple of favorite clubs, you've got plenty of material for inane conversations. The bar for conversations is really low. Given physical attraction, it takes a moderate amount of chitchat to then have sex. All you say is primarily filler, and the same applies to whatever she says.

Due to loud music it is difficult to have a proper conversation in a club anyway. Even in the quieter areas there is too much noise and distraction. Don't even try to have any kind of structured conversation. Make sure you get the info you need, like where she lives and who she is here with, and make sure you figure out some kind of commonality — it can be as simple as you both confirming that it's a great club you're in, or that you really enjoy living in your city. If in doubt, be a bit more positive than you otherwise might be. Again, it's not your verbal skills that get you laid in that kind of environment.

However, your verbal skills can easily *not* get you laid. I'm therefore going to give you some pointers regarding what to avoid talking about. Showing off your knowledge is generally a bad idea, because people — not just girls — normally don't enjoy that. Discuss your intellectual interests with your friends, fellow students, or colleagues, but not with people you hardly know. Likewise, it is a pretty bad idea to go into politics, religion, or sport, or any topic where you can expect most people to have strong opinions, even in the absence of any kind of critical thought as to why a certain position may be preferable over another.

If you are among the more educated, I would furthermore strongly advise you to restrain your vocabulary. Learn to talk like a normal person, at least for a few hours a day. A rule of thumb I found helpful was to avoid words I wouldn't expect a random teenager to know. This is not because I assume that you are going to focus on pulling teenage girls, but because the typical person is not terribly educated, even if they went to college.

A mistake I notice plenty of guys make is to show off achievements, particularly if they really have been successful in a particular area in their life. It's great that you've mastered X, whatever it may be, and I think that you should be proud of yourself, given that we live in a society in which the majority fills their spare time with unreflective media consumption. The woman you're talking to could have some particular interests, and if the two of you like each other a lot, you'll eventually learn about it. If she really is as shallow as she appears to be, you can still enjoy each other's company. It would be a shame if a pleasant sexual encounter went unrealized due to your immature posturing behavior.

Let me add that you'll find that the few ambitious and educated women, if they just want to get laid, tend to undersell their accomplishments and intellectual interests as well. I'm not convinced that college degrees are a good proxy for how smart or educated someone is. In fact, some of the biggest nonsense I've ever heard came out of the mouth of people with "expensive degrees", as they phrased it. Only very few pockets within higher education celebrate critical thinking and analysis. Most engage in little more than thinly-veiled indoctrination, intellectual circle jerks, and only let students think inside a slightly bigger box.

The dance floor

You don't need to be able to dance to pick up women on the dance floor, even though it can help. But before we get to this point, let's talk about how dance floors are normally structured. I'd like to think of them as having a periphery and a center. In the center you normally have people who dance in a much more expressive way. Sure, they may be drunk. If they are girls, then they mostly want attention. A much larger group of people at the periphery mostly goes unnoticed. They stand around or might move a little bit. You can tell that they don't feel overly comfortable in that environment.

I'm not going to talk about how to dance, and not just because this is difficult to describe in words. The much bigger reason is that dancing is often counterproductive. If you enjoy it, then I won't tell you not to, though. Yet, things will go much more smoothly, at least on a crowded dance floor, if you just walk around. You can approach women on the dance floor the same way you'd approach them at the bar, or on campus, or wherever else. If she's glancing over, and you walk up to her, then say something like, "Hey, how is it going?" If she was merely awkwardly stepping around, she'll quickly stop with those silly movements anyway.

On a very crowded dance floor you don't even have to dance. Instead, you calmly make your way through the crowd and watch out for women who are signaling that they want to be approached. Some may focus on you, others will make sure that men notice them. If you are in doubt, you can put a hand on her shoulder blade as you move through the crowd. I found this to be an excellent litmus test for how receptive a woman is. She doesn't even need to see you, as it's just a general response.

Some women will almost lean into you, revealing that they are basically looking for anyone. Of course, you have to meet certain minimum standards, but the early response is quite telling. This also works if you're directly approaching her and she sees you coming. In that case, though, you can probably gauge her interest by the way she's looking at you. Nonetheless, by touching her, you can quickly learn how physical she is.

Sexual escalation

Sexual escalation is a must if you want to get laid. However, the problem is that many guys go completely overboard. Once they've found a woman who wants them, they grope her in the most obscene ways and make out with her for half an hour or so. There are two problems with this approach. First, women can be very conscious of themselves, and she might not want to be seen acting like some slut in a night club in front of her friends or work colleagues. Second, sexual tension quickly dissipates if you give in too soon. By that I mean that women get more aroused if you only give in a little bit, because this will make them want you more.

To visualize this principle, think of how animals act. If you take your dog for a walk, and then suddenly give him some treats, he might do all kinds of tricks to please you and be very happy. Of course you can do it again and again, and again. But on the other hand, if you put a bag of treats on the ground and let him eat as much as he wanted, he would eat as much as he could. Once he has had enough, he might not bother much about performing tricks for you anymore.

Likewise, if you heavily arouse a woman, let's say you make out with her, and then you drag her into a dark corner and finger her to orgasm, she is likely to have gotten all the validation she was craving. In this example she not only got validation, but also a release for her sex drive. On the other hand, if you only kissed her for a little bit, and she started to get really horny, you could just say, "Let's get out of here!"

Don't view sexual escalation as some kind of routine you have to follow, though. Establish physical contact, ideally right when you approach her, and then take it from there. Rub her lower back, and maybe her ass. Some kissing is fine, too. I wouldn't go any further for the time being, at least if you don't intend to have sex inside the venue. Kiss for a little bit, and if you like how she does it, you can always suggest to continue this elsewhere.

You can't skip sexual escalation and think you'll just go through the motions once she is in your bedroom. In the rare case that you do get her there without much previous physical interaction, you'll find that she will be very uncomfortable about the idea of sleeping with you, and if you manage to turn her around, it will take you quite some time.

Another benefit of sexual escalation is that it establishes that she is interested in you. It's one thing for a girl to tell you that you're a seedy character and that she doesn't want to get involved with you, but quite another if she says this with a smile — right after she's been sucking on your neck. Further, it secures your position.

While there is always the chance that she'll move on to some hotter guy, this is virtually a non-factor if you established some physical contact. Talk to a girl for half an hour, but don't make a move, and she might keep looking around. Thus she's tempting other guys to approach her, and ditch you as soon as she can. On the other hand, if other guys have seen you kissing her, it is highly unlikely that they will interfere.

Physical contact shows your intentions, the stronger the sooner you establish it, and gives her an opportunity to decide whether she wants to continue with you. It communicates to her that you have a pronounced sexual interest in her, and because you did make a move already, she will not think that it is safe to talk to you for half an hour in order to appear more desirable to other suitors until someone better comes along.

How to be smooth

Some advice regarding sexual escalation seems in order, since guys are often doing it horribly wrong in clubs. Quite common is the bulldozer approach where guys go all out and put the woman in a potentially embarrassing situation, like going for a make out in front of her friends, when she has barely shown any sign of interest. This is obviously a bad idea. Instead, your level of sexual aggression should match her level of arousal. Of course, if she seems to be begging for it, you can rub her pussy, and in return put her hand on your crotch. Sometimes this happens moments after meeting her. All that's important is that you properly gauge her level of interest.

Sexual escalation is not a mechanical process where you start at literally zero, awkwardly touch her and pretend it was accidental, and after a long ordeal have sex with her. Instead, you react to her level of receptiveness. A girl that's dancing in a titillating manner, hoping to attract the attention of some guys, already signals that she's eagerly waiting for something to happen.

If you are unsure, you can always put your one hand on her waist and look deeply into her eyes. If she moves closer, presses her body against you, or stares at you, then she is only waiting for you to kiss her. This doesn't mean that you have to. All that matters is that she knows that you are willing and able to make a move, so one dominant gesture is normally sufficient to convince her that you are what women in romance novels always desire: a real man.

Squeeze her ass hard, or pull her hair a little bit, for instance. Both can be done in a very discreet manner, which some women find even more arousing. Pulling her hair discreetly might sound odd to you, but all it takes is that you put your hand firmly on her neck, move further up to her head, grab a hold of her hair and pull it down for a brief moment. This is often a huge turn-on. You shouldn't be afraid that this will go wrong because if she didn't want you to touch her, she wouldn't be standing so close to you and tolerate that you touch her neck.

The difference between merely making out with a girl

and getting laid often boils down to sexual escalation. Therefore, you have to learn to maintain sexual tension. Yes, even if she's touching your chest or squeezing your hard cock, you shouldn't lose control of yourself and tongue her down like a maniac. You won't be able to keep her very aroused for a prolonged amount of time, which means that she will eventually lose interest if you happen to arouse her too much too quickly. If you're standing at the bar, and the woman you're busy with is visibly horny and whispers into your ear that she can't wait for you to fuck her, then you have done something wrong if there is no way that you can quickly capitalize on that. In that case there is a good chance that you'll go home empty-handed.

By the way, if you find it difficult to keep her sufficiently aroused once you've kissed her, I'd recommend you not kiss her at all. Instead, be physical by holding her hand or pulling her in. Let her touch you, but don't kiss her. This builds up a lot of sexual tension, and if you nonetheless act quickly, it will be enough to get her to leave the venue with you. Smooth escalation is one thing, but to be really smooth, you would show very little overt physical affection, like making out with her, or biting her neck. Particularly, women who are past college age seem to appreciate a more discreet approach.

No matter how you decide to proceed, the key is to keep the tension. If you are too distanced, then she might question whether you are really interested. On the other hand, if you are too unrestrained, her passion will be gone as quickly as it has come. Seduction isn't a matter of how much time you've spent with her, but more a matter of opportunity and sexual compatibility. In order to leave the club with you, she has to find you sufficiently attractive.

However, she is probably willing to come home with you much sooner than you might think. Anything more than one hour is pushing it. I have had plenty of encounters where I, well, gained carnal knowledge of some girl within minutes of meeting her, thanks to unisex toilets or well-mannered bathroom attendants.

If I left the club with the girl, it was rare that it took me more than thirty minutes. It was often only ten or fifteen minutes before I said that it's about time we get out of here. This either resulted in giggling, a smile, or a coy look, which meant that I only had to take her hand and lead her to the coat check so that she could get her stuff.

A related issue is that you shouldn't be so dead serious when picking up girls. They go out to have fun, so even inappropriate behavior is encouraged, if you present a playful façade. For instance, if she looks at you seductively but seems to be interested in playing games, you could slap her ass to punish her. Even absurd maneuvers can work very well, like telling a girl who seems interested that you hope she doesn't mind if you check out her ass, followed by squeezing it while you keep talking to her. They giggle, tell you that what you are doing is inappropriate, but they nonetheless enjoy it, because they enjoy being desired by a man.

Taking Action

To lead means to be creepy

Women normally play a reactive role on the dating market in Western society. If you, as a guy, wanted to get laid without making any effort, you would need to be very good-looking or known to be wealthy, and even then most women still wouldn't make a move. The vast majority of guys do not have an enormous advantage over others in the dating market, and therefore have to look for girls who give off signals of general or specific interest, and approach them. Some women will turn them down, while others will welcome their advances.

Often girls realize that you may be interested in them, while they themselves aren't completely sure about it yet. Then they need to think about it, or consult with their friends whether you're really cool, because obviously she can't determine this for herself. More confident girls will, if they don't go home with you straight away, evaluate you and make a judgment based on how you present yourself. You'll notice that those tend to be a bit lukewarm towards you. Their mild approval of you can still lead to sex, but she might decide to wait for someone better to hit on her. According to persistent rumors there are even women out there who will try to get free drinks out of you before they walk off, or who will cock-tease because they like the feeling of being desired.

Some girls will flip from viewing you more neutrally to labeling you a creep — they might even loudly proclaim that you are one. Yes, you will not only receive polite rejections if you want to meet girls in the night life. Some girls are quite rude, in fact. Just smile, and maybe say to her that you're glad that she's saved you a lot of time, and move on. This might not be pleasant, but you will get used to it. Girls only call guys creepy if they don't find them attractive enough. If they like you, you can be more or less as bold and daring as you want. You're a creep not because of what you do, but merely based on whether the girl you hit on finds you attractive or not.

The best advice I can give you is to eliminate the word *creep* from your vocabulary. It's nonsensical. Let me rephrase this and instead say that it is situational. We guys don't use that word much anyway, but imagine you're at a bar and some mildly unattractive girl bumps into you, looks you in the eye, squeezes your ass and puts her lips dangerously close to yours. You're completely turned off by her behavior and want her to go away. But imagine that instead of some dog, it just so happened that a girl who looks like your favorite porn star walked in and has seemingly set her mind to fucking you. She's as aggressive as the other girl was, but suddenly you'd be much more appreciative and welcome her advances — at least until the alarm clock rings and you wake up.

It's better to pull her tonight

As you gather more experience in night clubs and bars, you'll learn not only that you have to focus on women who show some kind of interest, but also that some of them take a bit more time to pull than others. In some cases you part with a telephone number that will either flake or result in a date. If you are after sex, then this is the worst possible outcome, not just because your time investment will easily quadruple. It's also much more difficult to get a date than to have a one-night stand with a woman. I've written about this in the beginning of this book, in the section Benefits of clubs, but it's so important that I'll revisit this topic.

To the inexperienced, the statement that it's easier to have a one-night stand than to get a date sounds outlandish. To them a one-night stand is the pinnacle of seduction, which only the most experienced and suave men can pull off. But view it from her angle instead! If you meet her in a club or a bar, then, well, she is dolled up and away from her place already. She has made a significant investment of time, and she went to a club to have fun, as she would phrase it. This normally involves looking to meet some attractive guy. You're essentially a free bonus. You also have to consider psychological factors as well. If she is in the club, then she is in a much more adventurous and carefree mood. Thus, she is much more open to spontaneously having sex with some random guy.

Let's now contrast this to the dating scenario. If you meet her during the week, then she will spend some of her few hours of spare time. It may even be her only non-work related activity that day. As such, the time investment is quite substantial, so you'd better be a good prospect for a long-term relationship for her to consider meeting you, or fabulously handsome. Of course, it's also possible that she doesn't get much attention at all and is desperately waiting for some guy to make a move, but women in this category are pretty much by definition unattractive or undesirable.

The time investment is not just the time of the actual date. She now has to dress up just for you, and go all the way from her place to meet you somewhere, just for you. In addition, she is probably not in a particular mood to party and have fun, because she'll have another day of work or college ahead of her. It's not the weekend, after all.

From your perspective, the same reasoning applies. If you are going out anyway, and not only with the intention to hit on some broads, then sex with a random girl is essentially free, in the sense that the opportunity cost for taking a girl home once you are in the club is close to zero. Eventually you'll have to go home anyway, so why not take some girl with you?

The extended game plan

Without wanting to oversimplify things, there are only a few main cases on your nights out. In short, most girls you won't be interested in, and among those you are interested in, there are three possible scenarios:

- she needs a lot of time

- she only needs a pretense

- she's not interested

I know, I know, all women are different. But don't worry about that, because deep down they are all the same. If there is at least modest physical interest, and maybe a real or merely perceived lack of options, you are in a good position to get laid. This requires that you stick around, and it might also require talking a bit more than you would like to.

A common scenario is that you hit on a girl who is part of a group. You look presentable enough, and she doesn't want to look like a slut in front of her friends. The thought of exchanging phone numbers doesn't appeal to you because you know that her interest in you isn't particularly strong, which means that she'll quickly forget about you. On the other hand, you think that she's your best shot tonight, or that you don't want to leave the club or whatever.

Normally, you will then have to try to get accepted by her friends. The bigger the group, the less close they are anyway, so this might require nothing more than courtesy and an ability to conduct small talk. As long as you don't make any controversial statements or say anything that would require more than a second of thought, you'll probably be fine. If she didn't like you, she wouldn't want you to hang around anyway and either give you a strong hint that you aren't welcome, turn around and ignore you, or disappear to the bathroom for fifteen minutes to make you feel uncomfortable.

Hooking up in such situations is about endurance. In other words, if you don't get bored, it's a fairly safe bet. It is important that you manage to create some physical contact, for instance covertly holding hands, or having your arm around her waist. But do find out who she came with and how her friends relate to her. The less she knows them, the easier it will be to get her away from them.

Don't be indecisive, however. If you just stand around, enjoy some physical contact and chit-chat, then eventually the lights will come on, and she'll blurt out that she has to leave with her friends. Instead, spend at least some time alone with her. You could get drinks at the bar, go for a smoke, or catch some fresh air — or use this as a pretense to get her away from her friends and then suggest that she should get her coat.

A common scenario is that she and her best friend, naturally a girl, will have *the conversation*. She's unsure about you, so she discusses with her whether she should bang you. Sometimes girls are blatantly obvious about this. Your girl may tell you to wait for a moment. She then takes her girlfriend away, discusses excitedly what's going to happen — and if you're lucky, her friend, or possibly her entire group, either leaves without her or leaves you alone with her for a bit. You should view this as a green light, and a sign to not waste any more time. Get her out of there already!

Girls who need their sweet time can be a bit boring in bed, but you never know before you try anyway. While it's not my favorite situation, playing it safe and hanging around for an hour or so before making a move can work very well. It has the added side effect that you may make some new friends. This doesn't work so well if you only intend to have a one-night stand with her, or a short fling, but if she's part of a loose bigger social circle, and you go out in a somewhat tightly knit scene, you'll soon see your social circle expand, which will allow you to meet even more girls.

The efficient game plan

Maybe you don't always have a lot of time, or you simply want to maximize your chances. I mean, you could work on one girl the entire night, or you set yourself a limit of about half an hour before you move on. There is a good chance that in this alternative scenario you're leaving the club with the girl sooner than you would have gotten to first base with the other one.

The key is to very quickly move on to a physical level. Let's say some girl smiles at you. You then walk up to her and as you say hi, you don't stretch out your hand to formally introduce yourself, but put your arm around her waist and pull her close to you. This does require some experience since not all women will be comfortable with this. Don't push it if she seems to be a bit uptight. Assuming you have reached this level of experience, you then also know when to move the situation forward. Your bold opening move allowed you to instantly judge her reaction. What would you do if she pressed her body tightly against yours in response?

If she seems really into you, you can kiss her straight away. This works well in clubs and bars and, no, this doesn't mean that she is a slut. Most guys don't act like that, after all. Remember what I previously wrote about only approaching girls you are sexually interested in? This is why this is important, because by being physical you follow your desire, and your body communicates that you want her. Further, based on your experience you have judged her to be interested in you, so she will appreciate your bold move as well.

The goal is to establish a physical connection. Again, if the mere thought makes you feel uncomfortable, then take it a bit slower. Otherwise, do a bit of small talk. Make sure you don't ask any kind of interview questions but instead present yourself as the uncommitted kind of guy. If all of this goes well and she doesn't stop smiling at you, then take her somewhere else, say a quiet corner in the venue, so that you can talk to her.

Fondle her for a little bit but restrain yourself. You might find yourself finger banging her, in case things get hot and heavy, but if you get her off in the club she will probably be less interested in leaving with you. The same is true in the opposite case. If she finishes you off with her hands while passionately making out with you, then your level of sexual interest also quickly drops. If this is what you want, then go for it. Otherwise, stop her, ask her where she lives, so that you get this vital piece of information, and then leave with her.

You'll then probably hear her say that she is not that kind of girl or that she never does things like this, no matter whether this is true or not. If the two of you really can't restrain yourselves you can of course have a romantic encounter in a bathroom stall or in an alley. Otherwise, get a cab and make sure you keep her sexually aroused. This is a quite a thrill for her.

Depending on your personality, this style of picking up girls might not suit you, but if it does, and you find a girl who is really into you, try to accelerate all the steps you're already familiar with. You might be surprised how easy it can be to pull a girl home. Remember, what I just described can easily happen within 30 minutes. If you're starting out, aim for 45 minutes.

The incredible game plan

The previous two sections should give you all the information you need to successfully meet girls on your nights out. However, if you've read my book *Sleazy Stories*, or some other descriptions of my sexual encounters, you caught a glimpse of something even more extreme. Yes, it is possible to have sex with a girl within a few minutes in some dingy bathroom stall. No, this does not mean that you have to bribe her with coke — even though this seems to be a viable tactic in some circles.

When thinking of my successes, and when discussing them with a few guys who had similar experiences, I managed to distill the ingredients for rapid success. All of this takes some happy coincidences, and a significant amount of sexual experience on your part. The most important facet is that you are able to recognize whether she is really into you. If you still spend ten minutes pondering whether the girl that is sitting next to you on a bar stool and pressing her thighs against yours might be into you, then you are not quite there yet.

So, how does this work? I think it is indispensable that she is strongly attracted to you. Remember the early parts in this book where I wrote that you have to find your niche and stand out from the crowd? I don't think many women dream of having a one-night stand with Joe Generic, so do your homework. Apart from that, all that's needed is that she is sexually interested in you. Some girls need more time, and for those you should refer to the previous two sections. Other girls, though, are waiting to meet a guy like you. This implies initial interest. From there on you only have to feel out how ready she is.

You have to clearly communicate, non-verbally, that you won't waste her time. As I mentioned several times already, a common way for women to signal their interest is that they brush their tits against you as they walk past. You can quickly capitalize on this by grabbing her by the waist and pulling her in. As she then feigns surprise, you can basically say whatever you want. Just ask her how she's doing, while your lips graze her ear.

None of this implies that you are forcing yourself upon her. Being well-versed in seduction, you easily deduced from the way she looked at you that she finds you attractive. A little later you can normally make out with her. If you notice some resistance, then back off for a while. You don't have to take her home within fifteen minutes, after all. Yet, some women will get really turned on by a guy who is secure in himself and just goes for it.

It's not as if the clock is ticking and that you have to get laid as soon as possible, but at that point it's quite natural to move the conversation towards some dark corner. All you then have to do is capitalize on her momentary sexual interest. Make sure you figure out who she's with and where she lives. It's not as if you have to follow some kind of script, though. I've found that it worked remarkably well to simply get her to the point where she wants to make out with you, and then ask her where she lives.

She normally gets the hint. A simple, "Let's go!" is often all you need at this point. This suits her perfectly fine since she is horny already and can't wait to have sex with you.

Unfortunately, it might happen that she has to drive her friends home, catch an early flight the next morning, or show up to a job interview in six hours — all of those are stories I've heard myself. Amusingly enough, in all those cases the girls showed me plausible evidence, like an email on their smartphone, and they were bummed out that they couldn't spent the night with me. With the more adventurous ones, depending on your predilections, you can then suggest taking a walk that ends up in a nearby alley, or move the interaction to the bathroom stalls. The first option depends on the weather, and the second on an understanding bathroom attendant.

Picking the right spot

Okay, following my advice, you've got some girl hanging on your neck, and she's looking to score. What are you going to do with her? If your aim is merely to get laid, instead of trying to build some kind of connection, then you might want to consider the most convenient option. You can make out with her in any dark corner, and you'll easily get a hand job out of it. You can finger her, too. For anything more, dark corners are normally a dead end.

You could try taking her into a bathroom stall. In some clubs this is a no-go, either because the bathrooms are dirty, or because the attendant is over-eager and won't let you get down to business with some chick in one of *his* stalls. "Not in my stalls, buddy!", I once heard a bathroom attendant shout in my direction. You can always try bribing them, but then you're getting awfully close to directly paying for sex, which you may or may not like. In other venues you find spacious clean unisex bathrooms, without any bathroom attendants, that encourage sexual encounters.

In a bathroom stall pretty much anything goes. You can make out all you want, pull your cock out for a hand job, finger bang her. Blow jobs are normally a given. Sometimes, though, the toilet seats are gross, so she doesn't want to sit down, and squatting down in front of you may not always be so convenient. Oh, you can also fuck in a bathroom stall. For that to happen, though, you either lift her up on your lap, while sitting on the closed toilet seat, which is quite uncomfortable. Alternatively, you could turn her around, bend her over, and do her from behind. The problem with that, though, is that this can take quite a bit of energy, which you may not have in the early morning hours. For this to be somewhat enjoyable, she better not be too short, though. Well, here is another benefit of girls wearing high heels.

If the club isn't it, then head off to your or her place. It's perfect if you can walk there within a few minutes. Should you feel particularly adventurous, you can do the deed in a park or a dark alley, but this may lead to some unwanted attention if you choose the location poorly. Decide for yourself whether the thrill is worth it. I'd say it's a less interesting option than finding some suitable spot inside the venue.

In case your place is not within walking distance, you could take the bus or train, but this may turn into quite an odyssey. First, the journey may take a long time, and busses or trains often run very infrequently at night. Second, while she may have been super-horny and ready to jump your bone when she left the club, she will feel much less aroused if the two of you have to wait for the bus in the rain. Then there is the problem of having other people around. Some dude vomiting on public transport is a fairly reliable way to kill her mood. Loud crowds can likewise wreck an otherwise smooth pickup.

If you can afford it, I'd recommend getting a cab. It's fast and convenient, and you can basically start foreplay on the back seats. Head to your or her place. The eventual choice might depend on the cost and time, which in this case is synonymous. Surely you don't want to sit in a cab for 30 minutes when the other person lives a mere 10 minutes away. The advantage of getting back to your place is, well, that it's your place and you know where everything is. Of course, being a smart guy you keep your apartment clean enough. But even if you are a bit negligent with regards to your apartment, you know of bad surprises, if any. On the other hand, at her place anything could happen. Do you think you're going to get laid if she opens the door and her dog is lying on the carpet in his own vomit, because he ate the remains of the pizza she made ten days ago?

Especially among younger women it's quite common to have flatmates, which can make things more difficult as well. I once had it happen that, as I was about to mount some girl, the door opened and her completely drunk flatmate walked in, stark naked, and collapsed on the floor. She had taken a shower and apparently forgotten which one of the rooms in the apartment was hers. On the plus side, going home with girls will make you get to know your city better, in both good and bad ways. I've seen corners of London I would never have explored on my own, and I guess I can call myself lucky for never having been knifed or robbed, but that would be a story for another day.

Handling distractions

There is no sure thing in seduction, because a lot can go wrong. In this section I'm therefore highlighting some potential distractions, and how to deal with them. The starting point is that you have left the club and are on the way back to your or her place. Should you not have taken my advice of hailing a cab, I hope you were wise enough to stay away from loud groups on public transport. Make her focus on you. This is natural if you don't sit down but instead stand in some corner on the bus or train, and pull her close to you. Hold her, and kiss her occasionally. Make sure that you are standing in the corner, and she's facing you, so that she doesn't get visually distracted by other people.

Sometimes girls have the idea of getting something to eat on the way back because they are hungry. Don't go to any fast food joint and sit down. If she really has to have some crappy food early in the morning, make sure it's for a takeout. Tell her that you'd rather be at your or her place, spending time with her, instead of wolfing down a couple of cheeseburgers in that messy restaurant.

Once you're back at your or her place, don't drop the ball! She knows why she ended up alone with you, so move the interaction straight to the bedroom. You most certainly don't want to end up in a long conversation that makes the two of you forget what you came to the apartment for. You can have stimulating conversations with her after you've had sex, provided you're still interested in her then.

Sure, if she wants to have a glass of wine to loosen up a little bit, she should have it. This only applies if she's rather sober. What's likewise not okay is if she wants to sit down and eat. If she's stuffed, she won't quite feel like having sex. It might even make her more self-conscious, because she believes that she looks fat after eating something. Incidentally, this seems to be an issue much more common among very slim women. Feeling fat, she can't of course undress in front of you. Remind her with a smirk that food tastes better after sex.

What might happen is that she's not used to staying out

late, and is getting tired. Let's hope she isn't too tired to have sex. You should note that if she insists on you sleeping on the couch, you might as well pack your things and head back home. On the other hand, if she's still all touchy-feely, and says that she can't wait to bang you in the morning, then take proper precautions.

Imagine this scenario: she wakes up, it's bright, and she realizes that she's got a stranger sleeping in her apartment. Then she notices that her place is a total mess, and on top she's hungover. None of this is a great start for a sex session in the morning. Frankly, if she really wanted to have sex with you, her system would have been flooded with a cocktail of hormones that would have made her forget about her lack of sleep. Dopamine does that to people. But maybe she was just mildly interested. You can try preventing this situation by making sure that the curtains are all drawn before you lie down to sleep, because a darkened room will put her in a much more receptive mood than a brightly lit one.

Then there is the issue that you can't get it up. Yes, this happens to the best of us. Some guys keep a couple of boner pills in their back pocket for such situations, but it's not such a big deal either. Probably only virgin girls never had it happen that the guy couldn't get hard on command. Just don't feel bad about yourself or make excuses for it. You'll find it easier to perform the next morning, which girls know, too. She might even suggest going to bed and rest, with the more likely outcome that you spoon her, and that she'll do a little reach around to

check how your cock is doing, followed by some sponta-
neous sex.

On a related note, sometimes girls think it's their fault if
you can't get hard. Well, sometimes it is, like when she
attempts fellatio with teeth, which would kill any erection. If she's the kind of girl who does nothing like that,
but wants to blame herself, then take it easy. Tell her
that you're feeling tired, which is a quite legitimate reason after a night out, if you're not used to that lifestyle.
However, should this happen too often, then maybe reconsider some of your lifestyle choices.

Semi-successful attempts

You've tried your luck, but she's still a bit uptight. She
has no problem with you squeezing her ass, or making
out for a little bit, but she doesn't want to go home with
you. You've done everything you could, based on your
judgment. Now you could stick around until the end of
the night, but you know that this means gambling with
your time. Instead, prepare to move on. If you're in a
small club or bar, you might want to consider leaving the
place, because she won't view you favorably if she sees
you hitting on other girls. It will make her feel replace-
able, and women don't like that kind of feeling much,
even if they have a strictly physical interest in you.

No matter whether she is the kind of girl who needs a
lot of time for any guy who isn't completely her type, or

whether she didn't leave with you because her friends succeeded in preventing her from making some kind of mistake, as they would phrase it — all is not lost. After all, she found you attractive enough to enjoy your company for a while. If you want to continue with her, exchange contact details. Phone or message her the day after.

Do keep in mind that collecting numbers and hoping for a meet-up is fairly unreliable. If she was only mildly interested in the club, then it's highly unlikely that she'll want to hang out with you some later time. However, if there is a response, quickly suggest to hang out. This works quite well, and may lead to an easy lay. I don't recommend aiming for a date. You know her already and have spoken to her for maybe half an hour or so in the club already, and you can therefore continue from where you left off. Cook something at her place, have her come over to watch a movie or whatever. If she really has to meet up in a café beforehand, pick one that's close to your place.

Some girls may suggest that you meet her and her girl-friends at some bar before they move on to a club. This a great idea if you are keen on wasting your time, and don't mind not getting laid yet again. In the worst case you are in for another long night, and who says that you'll get her this time? Her friends might interfere once more and tell you that she is tired or has a lot of stuff to do the next day or some other bullshit excuse. You only want to meet her alone. As a compromise, you can invite her to your place, and after you've had sex, you can drop her off at wherever her girlfriends are meeting, if it's on the way.

Cutting your losses

As you gain more experience, you'll realize that you've got many more options than you initially thought. While you might not get laid every weekend, it's not such a rare occurrence, and you aren't afraid of having another dry spell, being fully aware that it's basically a matter of time until you'll get laid again. This is an important insight that leads to a much more laid-back attitude towards dating. There is no need to desperately make every interaction count. Yes, if you are into her, and she's into you, make the most of it. On the other hand, trying to get laid with women who are hardly interested in you is something you'll hopefully drop at this point.

The problem is that while it sometimes may happen that she hasn't many options and lets you stick around in case nobody better comes along, it could as well happen that after a time investment of two hours or more, which were as tedious for you as for her, she eventually walks off. The best outcome would have been sex devoid of all passion, so even turning such an interaction around is a waste of time. The payoff of such interactions is unbelievably bad. It's either wasting a few hours and getting nothing, or wasting a few hours and getting bad sex.

If the interaction is a drag, and she seems hardly interested, but for whatever reason tolerates you, I'd recommend you move on. It's simply not worth it. Instead,
hit on other girls who are potentially much more interested in you, and with whom you know after maybe half
an hour how your chances are. You should want to either get approval, or disapproval, but not some vague
non-committal behavior.

Making it a lifestyle?

I won't recommend that you devote your twenties or
thirties exclusively to pulling ass from the club. However, there probably will be times in your life when you
want to get laid a bit more often. For some guys this happens after college, when they get their first real job and
have money to spend. Or maybe your wife divorced you
for whatever spurious reason, and you're still in a good
age for pulling girls. In any case, if you are serious about
this, then you should live reasonably close to the clubs
and bars you like.

It is fantastic if you live within walking distance. Imagine how easy it would be to get laid if your apartment
was ten or fifteen minutes away. You could easily take
a girl home, bang her, and bring her back to her fake-
concerned friends before the club closes. You may have
to make some trade-offs regarding rent or the condition
of the building. But even if it's a dingy room, it's no problem. As long as you keep it clean, you'll be fine. Don't

worry about the size either. An apartment close to the party district of your city might be a bit more expensive, so you'll have to lower your expectations a little bit.

There is also a great psychological benefit to living close to the clubs, namely that you won't talk yourself out of going out, since the time investment is minimal. On the other hand, if you lived in the suburbs and weren't quite sure whether you wanted to head out, you'd probably stay in. In the worst case, you'd always find an excuse not to go out.

For those of you who are less keen on partying three or four times a week, make some adjustments to your monthly budgeting. Spending money on a cab, or a hotel room, can make the difference between you getting laid and walking home with blue balls. If you live rather far away, it would take a lot of trust from her to go home with you. On the other hand, following you into a hotel will probably make her feel a lot less uncomfortable.

Keep going!

We've covered a lot of ground. Let me now give you some last guiding words before we part. The material in this book might take some time to sink in. You might have to make a significant effort to improve yourself, and possibly even change aspects of your personality, which isn't easy. However, I am confident that if you take the material in *Club Game* seriously you will see some success. You don't have to aim to have sex with as many women as possible, or as quickly as possible. Instead, try to figure out what you want to get out of all of this.

Don't forget to have fun while you go out! While it's enjoyable to interact with women, and take them home, the main purpose of going to a club or bar should be that you like being there. You should like the atmosphere, the music they're playing, and the people who go there — or at least a few of them.

With some guys there is an element of narcissism involved when it comes to picking up women. They want to make things more difficult for themselves by picking up girls in a place they don't fit in, or they want to learn how to pick up girls in all kinds of environment. Such challenges might be inherently satisfying. However, I don't think you should define yourself by the number of women you manage to pull home, or how allegedly difficult it was. It's okay if things are easy. You want to get laid with girls who are into you, not with those you have to convince, don't you?

I would like to encourage you to keep going until you find something that works for you. From that point onward you'll only have to iterate. Once I had found a clothing style that worked for me, I threw out some of the other stuff I bought. Thankfully, I had discovered a more or less timeless style that served me very well for years, and did not require me to spend much time on fashion research, or much money on updating my wardrobe. I replaced worn-out pieces, or got similar ones.

Likewise, once I had found a scene in which I had great success with girls, and with the kind of girl I was interested in, I kept at it. There was plenty of variety to be had, I had great fun, and the fact that it was comparatively easy for me to get laid didn't mean that my interactions were devalued in any way.

Of course you can do whatever you want, but consider experimenting only until you find something that seems to work for you, and in your environment. Afterwards, you should focus on refining your outfit, and streamlining your interactions. If you get to that point, you will have successfully integrated club game into your life, and you will find yourself in the comfortable position of being able to easily meet new women.